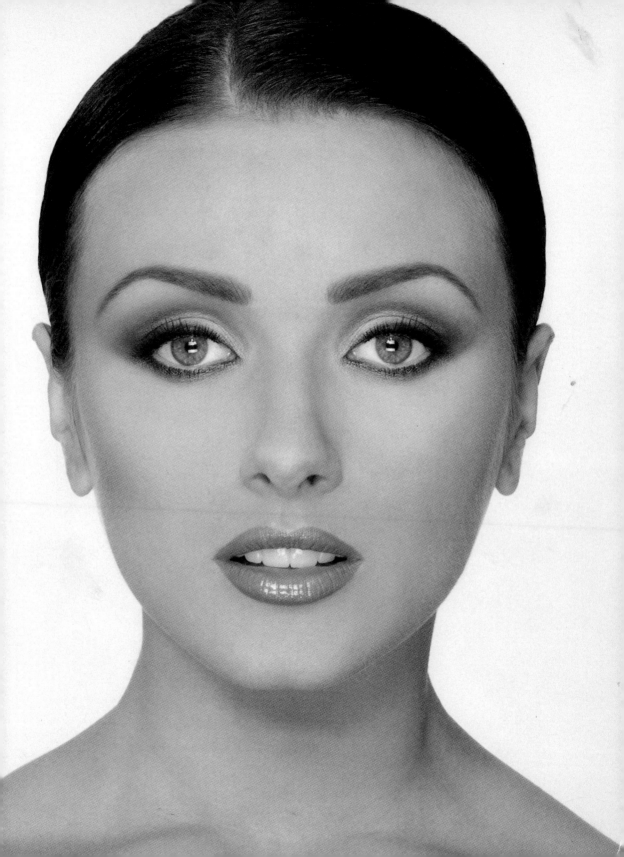

Plastic Surgery Without the Surgery

The Miracle of Makeup Techniques

Eve Pearl

EMMY AWARD–WINNING CELEBRITY MAKEUP ARTIST

WARNER BOOKS

An AOL Time Warner Company

Warner Books, Inc., 1271 Avenue of the Americas, New York, NY 10020
Visit our Web site at www.twbookmark.com.

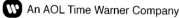 An AOL Time Warner Company

Printed in the United States of America
First Printing: January 2004
10   9   8   7   6   5   4   3   2   1

Library of Congress Cataloging-in-Publication Data
Pearl, Eve
    Plastic surgery without the surgery : the miracle of makeup techniques / Eve Pearl.
        p. cm.
    ISBN 0-446-53169-3
    1. Beauty, Personal. 2. Cosmetics. 3. Skin—Care and hygiene. I. Title.

RA778.P3146 2003
646.7'26—dc21

2003052590

Principal photography by Robert Milazzo.
Still lifes photographed by Alex Kroke.
Design by Platinum Design, Inc., NYC, and HRoberts Design.

This book is dedicated to:

My mother, Riva, who has been my inspiration, support, and role model my entire life.
As an immigrant coming into this country, she taught me to never be afraid of anything and that the
world holds endless possibilities for us all, at any age.

My son Joseph, for always being by my side and my motivation.
Whose amazing creative, technical, visual, and audio talent I couldn't do without.

My husband, Todd, for his incredible love and support.
Who has always believed and encouraged me to pursue my dreams.

The wonderful women who gave of themselves, their time, face, and body.
Without them, I would not be able to show that we are all beautiful women.

The incredible people I work with who stood by me through it all.
Thank you for your strength, your support, and believing in me.

Acknowledgments

I would like to extend much gratitude:

- To Billie Fitzpatrick, my collaborator, who took my words and thoughts and translated them into a flowing whole.

- To my incredible editor, Diana Baroni, whose caring support, professionalism, and guidance made this magnificent experience with this project possible. To everyone at Warner Books, especially Molly Chehak, Tina Andreadis, Flamour Tanuzi, Penina Sacks, and Tom Whatley. To Howard and Helen Roberts at HRoberts Design for your creative style.

- To my fantastic photographer, Robert Milazzo, whose talent, generosity, and endless positive energy made this experience a joy. To Alex Kroke, whose precision, skill, and patience are priceless. To the team at Robert's studio, Dan Engel and Thomas Chu. To Adrian Velez for your beautiful illustrations.

- To my amazing team: Melanie Demitri, my utmost respect goes out to you as my trusted right hand and makeup assistant. Maria Ponsiano, my second makeup-and-everything-else assistant. John Monroe, for your hairstyling. Deirdre Flaherty, for being my hairstylist and a terrific friend. Erma Eliazov, for your brilliant fashion styling for all ages. Tiffany Hodges, for meticulously completing my vision. Jennifer Bissu, for your illustrations. Dan Welch, for your enthusiasm and an eye to capture everything on tape. Deborah Hetrick for your troubleshooting help.

- To Randy Rahm for your generosity with your incredible fashion designs. To Julie Alderfer for your continued fashion help both on and off air. To Marty Melik and Jacqie Ogle for always coming through.

- To the amazing women who gave their time, face, and body for this project: Amy K. Browne, Podessa Ross, Colleen Gilson, Shirley Sutherland, Gillian Murphy, Doris Rhodes, Riva Pizhadze, Rachel Spiller, Tamara Pizhadze, Elena Cristiean, Claudia Zahn, Sung Yun Lee, Tiffany Walton, Kimberly Cull, Iteka Oldwine, Barbara Geddie, Mary McDonah, Deirdre Flaherty, and Maia Guest.

- To Irina Dvorovenko, Maria Bencebi, Victoria Carollo, Ashley Alderfer, Katlin Sotel, Danita Chantel, Maria Ponsiano, Deirdre Cossman, and Julia Wang.

- To Helene Godin and Nancy Wolff, whose caring professionalism and guidance made this project possible. To Ernest Gary, for your organization.

- To my mom and dad, Riva and Misha; my husband, Todd; my boys, Joey, Tucker, and Sterling and my brother, Michael. To my extended family and friends, Rudy, Doris, Marc, Irma, Lisa, Joe, Jill, Nazi, Repico, Alex, Svetlana, Emeda, Yuri, Susan, Yura, Marina, Ester, Fred, Jeffrey, Bryan, Yelena, Connie, and George.

- A special thanks to Meredith Vieira: You are that ray of sunshine that reminds us all that there are incredible people in this world. I feel blessed for the privilege of working with you. You raise the bar and show us it's possible to achieve our goals and still be a wife, mother, and friend. And to the "PP" (Deirdre Flaherty, Amanda Wessels, Fran Taylor, and Alison Frances).

- A special thanks to Kelly Ripa: You are a genuinely beautiful person, both inside and out. You encourage us all to reach for the stars, obtain them, and still keep our feet on the ground and our priorities straight. Kimberly Jason, thanks for your assistance.

- To the incredible people I've had the honor to work with on a daily basis for many years: Bill Geddie, Barbara Walters, Joy Behar, Star Jones, Lisa Ling, Debbie Metenopolous, Marcy Walker, Mark Gentile, Dusty Cohen, Joyce Carollo, Richard Esposito, Linda Menching, Anne Michelle Radcliffe, Robin Kaiser, Robert Baker, Suzy Alvarez, Judy Chin, Tom Molinelli, Barbara Simmons, Victor Callegari, Tatiana Zinovoy, Chris Mauro, Susan Haber, Richard Monge, Marque, Lorie Klein, Bryant Refroe, Elena George, Lavette Slater, Linda Finson, Jessica Stedman Guff, Randy Barone, Penny Hageanon, Jack Burrows, Susan Solomon, Donald Berman, Patrick Ignozzi, Jakki Taylor, Glenn Davish, Haleigh Safran-Raff, Audrey Jones, Matt Strauss, Dana Goodman, Karl Nilsson, Rob Bruce-Baron, Phyllis Digilio, Rob Naylor, Colleen Marquis, Gerry Donnelly, Brooke Kalick, Rachel Giordano, Lauren Mack, Amy Ryder, Rita Ienco-Plaza, Diane Trafford, Emily Coons, Natalie Bubnis, Lauren Brennan, Alina Perez, Shannon Walker, Allison Storelli, Christian McKiernan, Andrew Smith, Rich Provostt, John Keegan, Dvorah Rabino, Michael Spiteri, Candice Dunn, Robert Caufield, Harold Hernandez, Jason Kornblatt, Justin Montanino, Angela LaGreca, Bo Dronyak, Tom Egan, Dave Gavagan, Bill Mickley, Brian Connelly, Scott Lanchenauer, Ken Egan, Kevin Egan, Tim Shea, Rene Butler, Roger Williams, Jared Heinke, Tangie Valmon, Rich Freedman, Frank Cocchia, Russ Fortier, Trever Thompson, Ed Garofalo, Marvin Bronstein, Nick Caputo, Horace Eccleston, Sonya Coleman, Mary O'Leary, and Ayesha Johnson.

Contents

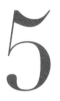
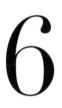

Introduction

When a woman hits a certain age, it's only natural to consider some type of cosmetic surgery. Women feel so much pressure to resist aging that they begin to look for anything possible to make them look and feel younger. Unfortunately, many of these women turn too quickly to plastic surgery: Two and a half *million* cosmetic surgeries are performed each year in the United States alone, one-quarter of which are done on women under the age of twenty—and that number continues to grow. Why do so many women want to change their looks? The constant barrage of media representations of abnormally thin and beautiful models makes most of us feel less than perfect, causing us to question our looks instead of accept them. A woman recently said to me, "As a girl, I was terrified to grow up. I would look at the magazines and say, 'I don't look that way. How will I be happy? Have a boyfriend? Will people like me?' My whole world seemed to depend on me looking like the cover girl models."

Such is the pressure created by airbrushed perfection. We know that these images are false and misleading, but we also know they are not going to go away. So what do we do? Many women turn to an array of cosmetic surgery procedures—from face-lifts to eye lifts, Botox, breast augmentations, and more. The procedures, however, are not only expensive, but also risky and sometimes quite dangerous. A California plastic surgeon recently attributed the rising rate of botched operations to improper training of surgeons. Over the past four or five years, he has seen a 20 to 30 percent increase in requests to redo such botched jobs. Plastic surgery is not the only answer. In fact, in my opinion, there is a better, safer, easier solution. It's the oldest trick in the book, and the technique that is used for those "perfect" models on magazine covers and for celebrities on television and in film: makeup.

I spent years creating faces as a makeup artist for theater on Broadway, in the opera, and in the ballet. Since then, I have been working with celebrities on television and film as well as doing photo shoots, yet I still cling to the makeup techniques I learned in the theater. I've realized that many of the tools and strategies for making a face come alive onstage remain the same in everyday life, though not to such dramatic degrees. In the theater, I learned an important lesson about the dual powers of makeup and the naked face:

Every face is a blank canvas, and makeup can easily alter and augment facial characteristics, constructing dimension in a variety of ways. The techniques are simple and create amazing results. They are the reason why models and celebrities always appear flawless. In this book, I will reveal these secrets, so you can look (and feel!) flawless, too.

No matter what we do or where we live, we all sometimes feel judged by the way we look. My mother, who I feel is beautiful, is constantly agonizing over whether or not she should cave in to the pressure and get a face-lift. Her fears of the pain and of the results have kept her away from the surgeon, along with some simple makeup techniques I showed her that "lift" her face. Now she can look younger every day—without the risks or the cost of surgery. Like many women, I personally struggled with the way I look, and I've been known to obsess about my acne scars—especially since I work in an industry where it feels as though you are constantly judged by the way you look. Even the most beautiful—and young—women suffer from some insecurity over what they see as imperfections in how they look, whether it's an occasional breakout, puffy eyes, or a double chin. All of these so-called problems can be fixed with makeup. Keep in mind that the appeal of a beautiful woman is also her sense of humor (think of Lucille Ball), her intelligence (Eleanor Roosevelt), her poise and elegance (Jackie O), her confidence (Catherine Zeta-Jones), her drive (Madonna), her longevity (Elizabeth Taylor), and, at times, her vulnerability (Princess Diana). Without a doubt, beauty is a subjective quality, but one that we all strive for to some degree. Makeup gives each and every woman the power to find her particular beauty, and this power is the true value of makeup.

I wrote this book because I wanted to share with others what I have discovered over the past fifteen years working as a makeup artist. Of the many people whom I have helped get ready for the camera, all have said one thing consistently: "I didn't know makeup could do that!" They were amazed at the power of certain techniques to transform their faces, their eyes, their brows, their noses, their lips, and other aspects of their bodies.

I also want to share these secrets as a way to empower women (and men)—especially as a defense against the omnipresent cultural pressure to have the "perfect" face and body. In this day and age, when it seems as if everyone is considering some form of surgery or other interventional procedure to "correct" their face or body, makeup is a powerful, safe way to enhance your appearance and alter those features that you want to change without complication. Makeup is both inexpensive and temporary, two qualities that are decidedly not characteristic of plastic surgery. We invest time and money in gyms (we never go to), diet programs (we don't stay on), shopping for clothes (we never wear). Why not invest some time into making ourselves feel better about ourselves? Applying makeup is quick, easy, and fun. Learning how to use it to temporarily accentuate or completely transform your face is quite simple—just follow the guidelines in the pages that follow. I promise, you'll be amazed by the results!

In the first chapter, you will learn about your skin type and how to choose the right foundation, as well as other makeup products that best suit your skin type. We'll then move on to the face. You will see how to use makeup to lift your face or forehead, hide those freckles, enhance your cheekbones, remove that double chin, and more. In chapter 3, you'll learn how to accentuate or deaccentuate the eyes and brows, as well as hide those dark circles, puffy eyes, and crow's-feet. Contemplating eyelid surgery? No need. I'll show you how to get the same effect with makeup. Chapters 4 and 5 discuss the nose and lips. Forget that nose job or Botox to enhance your lips—you can create the nose and lips you want in only a few simple steps. In chapter 6, we'll look at the breasts and the body, focusing on how to make your breasts look fuller (you won't believe your eyes!) and how to temporarily hide unwanted age spots or tattoos. Finally, in chapter 7, you will find an overview of all the makeup tools you'll need to transform yourself. In addition, throughout the book, you'll discover tons of unique home remedies, beauty tips, and tricks of the trade that will also enhance your look.

So forget the risky and expensive procedures and surgeries! Makeup not only lets you hold on to the part of yourself that your unique face represents, but also gives you the power to discover all the people you want to be. Let makeup be your magic wand!

Plastic Surgery Without the Surgery

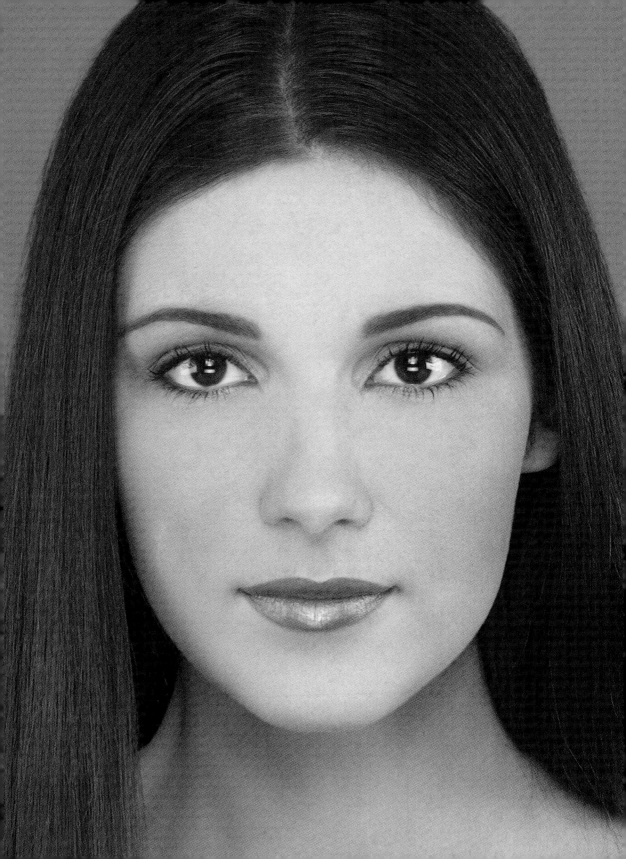

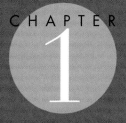
your
skin
SO SOFT, SO REAL

Our face is our canvas. Until we reach our thirties, our skin is able to renew and maintain itself quite easily. But as we get older, we need more help to maintain its health and appearance. Between not drinking enough water, the stress of daily life, poor diet, and the effects of the environment—including sun and wind, not to mention the indoor hazards of ultraviolet light, poor air circulation, and drying heat—we wreak havoc on our skin. Thankfully, we can do a lot to help recharge and rejuvenate our largest organ through the creative use of makeup. But before we get to the various tips for transforming your face, eyes, nose, and lips in the following chapters, we must determine what kind of skin you have.

Understanding Your Skin Type

Our skin, like the weather and our moods, does change. Rarely will you always be dry or oily. Changes in weather, diet, or menstrual cycle can cause your skin to feel drier, oilier, or even more acne-prone. Having said that, however, most of us do tend to experience some sort of combination skin, being prone to having dry or oily skin the majority of the time.

OILY SKIN

Those of us with oily skin don't appreciate the fact that oil production helps maintain a youthful look and keeps us wrinkle-free longer than most. All we see is that shiny nose, the glowing forehead, and the shadow of another zit ready to surface. As we try to dry out the oils by using harsh, drying cleansers and applying products with alcohol to strip away the shine, we achieve a temporary oil-free, matte-finish effect. In the long run, however, this actually exacerbates the situation, by causing the sebaceous glands of the skin to produce even more oil. Those of us with oily skin should consider these products and follow this advice:

- Use a pH-balanced toner or a regular cleanser.
- Buy an oil-free moisturizer and do continue to moisturize.
- Try an oil-free or matte-finish foundation.
- Avoid eye shadows that are dewy or contain too many shimmers; instead of having the desired effect, they can cause you to look a bit oily.
- Apply loose face powder to set foundation and keep it in place.
- When your face is shiny, use oil-absorbing blotting papers or pads, which absorb the oil without leaving behind another layer of powder.
- Along with applying foundation, use an anti-shine product available in a gel tube or other container, which can be applied before or after foundation. An anti-shine can also be applied along your hairline and on your scalp to absorb oil. It is colorless, goes on wet, and dries up. Think of it as a type of antiperspirant for your face.
- Use powdered blush and eye shadows. Cream blushes and eye shadows might have a tendency to get blotchy and mush together.
- Thin out your foundation by moistening a makeup sponge with water, patting it dry, and then applying foundation.

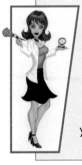

For a Shiny Nose

If you're at an event and you feel your face getting oily, instead of pulling out the compact and powdering over the oil, try to first use your napkin (hopefully it's clean) to dab off excess oil. You can also use a tissue, toilet paper, or cloth. This will prevent the layering of oil and powder on your face and keep your skin from appearing shiny.

COMBINATION SKIN

I believe most of us fall into this category. Our skin tends to be oilier in the T-zone (the area across our forehead and down the nose to the chin), but dry around the edges. Combination skin creates confusion among women since we are not sure if we should continue to moisturize or not—especially in spots where our skin is oily. Remember, whether we have dry or oily skin most of the time, we all need to moisturize around our eyes and lips to prevent those crow's-feet (wrinkles) from developing. Here is some advice for combination skin:

- Use gentle cleanser.
- Buy liquid or cream foundation.

- Use powder blush and eye shadow.
- Blotting papers are great as a touch-up for absorbing oil.
- Continue to moisturize all over your face. Apply a thinner coat in oilier areas. There are also many oil-free moisturizers that can hydrate your skin.
- Change moisturizers every now and then; this will rejuvenate your skin and increase circulation.

SENSITIVE SKIN

Many of us have experienced an unpleasant reaction to skin products at one time or another. Those of us with sensitive skin must be diligent in our search for hypoallergenic cosmetics in order to prevent skin reactions from occurring. Here is some general advice for those with sensitive skin:

- Avoid products containing fragrance, live plant extract, lanolin, or alcohol.
- "Fragrance-free" does not mean allergen- or chemical-free. Check the label.
- It is important to consider your skin type. If you have dry skin, you should avoid oil-free and oil-absorbing makeup, which will give your skin a parched, flaky finish. For those with oily skin, avoid moisturizing makeup that will make skin look slick and greasy. Normal skin types should stick with a makeup formulated for normal skin.

No Woman Can Do Without It: Moisturizer

Everyone can use a little moisturizing, and it's important to moisturize your insides as well as your outside. How do you take care of those vital organs? Drink plenty of water! Not only does water help eliminate the natural toxic buildup in all the organs and tissues of your body, but it also helps keep your skin hydrated. In addition, using a topical moisturizer at least once daily will also help to keep your skin feeling moist and healthy. When you choose a moisturizer, keep these things in mind:

- Check the labels. There are oil-free water-based moisturizers for oily skin (noncomedogenics—to prevent breakouts) and water-in-oil moisturizers for dry skin. Use the moisturizer that best fits your skin.
- You might want to try a thicker cream in the evening, especially around the eyes. Please note that when I say *thicker*, I don't mean to glob it on. Use a heavy cream, but apply it sparingly around the eye area using only your fingertips, gently dabbing it on. Otherwise, it will not be absorbed; your eyes will actually look puffy in the morning. Even those of us with oily skin should use a thick cream, especially in delicate areas around the eyes. Everyone needs extra moisture. Many people with oily skin, myself included, have tried to dry out their skin, making it much worse. Since I've been using a thicker cream, however, my skin just feels more nourished, instead of more oily. You can even use a thick oil-free moisturizer.
- Don't forget the neck! Many of us neglect this delicate area, but it needs moisture, too. The skin is thin and can give away our age if not properly maintained.

- During the day, try a light moisturizer. If you apply moisturizer on a slightly damp face, it will thin out and go on much more sheer.
- The sun can be very dangerous to the skin. Try using either a moisturizer or foundation with sunscreen.
- If you're using an anti-shine product, apply it after the moisturizer.

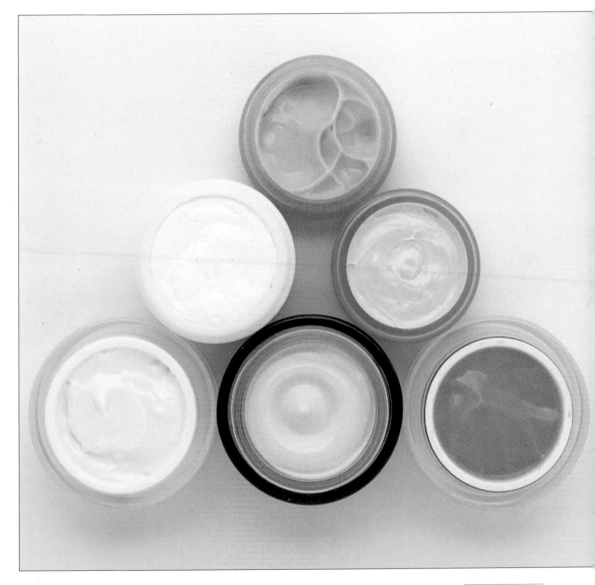

How to Choose and Use Foundation

- First, you need to decide how much coverage you need. Sheer foundations are good for a light, natural coverage. Moderate coverage is a good choice for those of us with some discoloration, a few acne scars, and maybe some freckles or broken blood vessels. Heavy- or full-coverage foundations offer the most camouflage. They're good for covering burns, birthmarks, bruising, melasma, and scars.
- We've all grown up seeing women (including ourselves) testing the shade of a foundation on the back of the hand. When was the last time you held up your hand to your face? The two are rarely the same shade. The best place to test the color of a foundation is on the side of your face, between your cheek and jawline. Your goal when you apply the foundation on the lower part of your face is to find the color that appears the same shade as your neck. We've all seen women with a face one shade and the rest of the body a different shade. (Some of us have even been those women.) This could mean that you need to adjust your foundation in the summer and winter. Remember, although your face is your canvas, it's still attached to the rest of your body.
- Caucasian women have a tendency toward red pigmentation in the face, which is why they flush and their skin can become red and blotchy. They need a foundation with some yellow pigment to balance out the redness. Stay away from pink or orangey tones.

Quick Tips to Combat Dry Skin

- Drink plenty of water.
- Use cream moisturizers.
- Mix moisturizer with concealer when applying around the eye area to prevent creasing.
- Choose a moisturizing oil-based foundation (silicone).
- Lightly powder with a brush.
- Use cream or powder blush.
- Using shimmers on your face and eyes will help give a dewy look.

- Mediterranean, Latin, and Asian women tend to have a more olive tone to their skin. Olive-, beige-, or neutral-toned foundations with a yellow undertone work best.
- African American women have a tendency to have oilier skin, which can turn the foundation darker than it first looked on the skin. These women need to choose shades a bit lighter than the skin, and to stay with warm honey tones. Avoid overly yellow or olive shades, which can turn ashy and gray after being applied.
- The most important thing to remember when choosing a foundation is to match the foundation to your skin tone. The descriptions above are a general guideline.
- Foundation can be applied with the fingers, with a makeup sponge, or both. Dot liquid foundation on your T-zone (across the forehead, then down and around the nose to your chin) and, using your fingers or a makeup sponge, blend the makeup out toward the hairline, cheeks, and jawline. If you're using a cream or wet-to-dry foundation, glide a makeup sponge along the foundation to get a light coating and apply to the T-zone area, while blending outward.
- When applying foundation, don't forget to blend down to your neck. (It should match the color of your neck.)
- When buying products at a cosmetics counter, carry a mirror with you. Go outdoors and check your face with your neck before making a purchase—that's the true test.
- When applying foundation, don't forget your eyelids, the corners of your nose, and your lips.
- After applying foundation, if you feel that there might be too much on, simply blot with a tissue. This will eliminate excess oil or moisture from the foundation.
- Try not to get stuck with using the same color or texture for your foundation all year round. Your skin changes with the seasons. At times it's dry or oily. It also gets slightly darker or redder in the summer, then paler in the winter. Try to adjust your makeup to your skin.
- During summer months, you might need to add some color to your neck and under your chin. It's the one area that seems to miss the sun—so your face and chest might end up one shade, and your throat area another. Usually, I suggest matching your face to your neck. In these cases, however, try to apply a blush or bronzer to your neck area.
- Try experimenting with different products. We sometimes spend more time shopping for things we put on our feet or under our clothes than we do for products that go right on our faces.
- Create a flawless canvas with foundation or concealer and everything that follows will look better.

Hands

Many of us take great care of our faces but forget our hands. They are a sure giveaway to our age. They are always out there in the sun, water, and wind, enduring harsh chemicals and doing our hard work. They are prone to sun and liver spots, wrinkles, puffiness, and dryness.

- Apply excess face moisturizer on your hands.
- Always moisturize your hands after washing them, especially in the winter.
- Apply excess hand cream on your neck, elbows, and legs.

COMMON PROBLEM AREAS AND THEIR COLOR SOLUTIONS

BODY AREA	ISSUE/PROBLEM	LIGHT/MED SKIN	MED/DARK SKIN
Undereye	Bluish veins	Light peach/salmon	Honey yellow/salmon/orange
Undereye	Red/bluish (looks purplish)	Yellow/light peach/salmon	Honey yellow/salmon
Undereye	Dark brown/reddish	Yellow/light peach	Honey yellow/salmon
Face/body	Acne—red	Yellow	Honey yellow
Face/body	Acne—brown/black	Yellow	Honey yellow/salmon
Face/body	Freckles—brown/raised black	Yellow	Honey yellow
Face/hands	Sun/liver spots	Yellow	Honey yellow/salmon
Neck/body	Hickey/bruise/tattoo	Yellow/light peach	Honey yellow/salmon

Avoid using white or shades that are too light to cover up an area.

This will usually turn ashy or chalky—and instead of disguising the area,

it will draw attention to it.

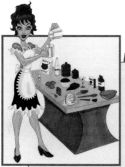

- **Vitamins:**
Vitamin E, A, or C capsules (in gel form), from your local drugstore, can be used instead of the costly creams with these ingredients in them. Prick open the capsule and add its contents to your moisturizer. You'll get all the benefits of the expensive creams without the extra chemicals or expense.

- **Baking soda:**
Mix three-quarters of a cup of baking soda with one-quarter cup of water, gently rub on your face for three minutes, and rinse off. A great, inexpensive exfoliator.

- **Hydrogen peroxide:**
Apply with a cotton ball. Makes a terrific astringent.

- **Pepto-Bismol:**
A great face mask for sensitive skin. The same way it coats and soothes the stomach, it gently caresses the skin. Apply straight from the bottle with a cotton ball. Allow it to dry and rinse with cool water. It's soothing and refreshing.

- **Vodka and lemon:**
Tone up tired skin by mixing a quarter cup of vodka with the juice from one lemon. Dab this on your face, neck, and chest area with cotton. Not necessary to rinse off. It will evaporate with the air. The less rubbing, the better. Mix a bit extra (with some sugar) and have a cocktail.

Now that you are familiar with some of the basics, you are ready for more tricks of the makeup trade. In the next chapter, Facial Magic, you will see how several women of all ages and looks transform their faces in quick and easy steps.

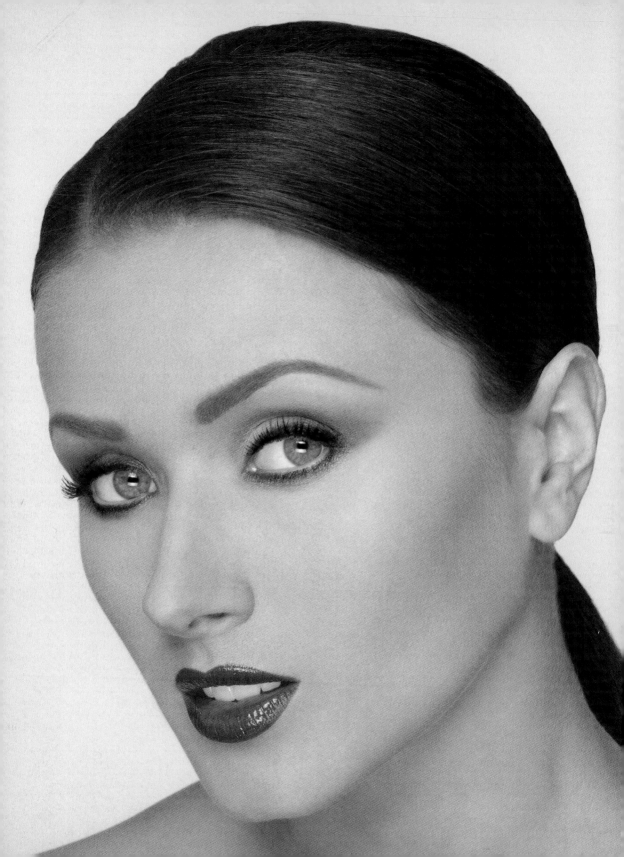

facial
magic
HIGHLIGHTING YOUR OWN
SPECIAL BEAUTY

Beauty—be not caused—It Is—
Chase it, and it ceases—
Chase it not, and it abides—
Emily Dickinson

Each of us possesses a unique face. This uniqueness is an important part of our identity, our signature, and sometimes even our armor. And yet most of us have at one time or another wished we could somehow change the face with which we were born, or erase the signs of aging we have developed over the years. Instead of admiring our distinctive features—a high brow, an aquiline nose, prominent cheekbones, deep laugh lines, a dimpled chin—we tend to bemoan what we see in that mirror.

The truth is, we all want to *feel* beautiful. But how do we get to that place in which *feeling is believing*? More important, how do we accept our uniqueness in the face of the constant pressure to look similar to the models, actresses, and beauty queens who inundate the magazines? And by the way, they don't start out looking like that. Let me share one secret: It takes hours of makeup, hair, lighting, and usually computer retouching to achieve the effect of perfection in the women—both young and old—who appear on the covers of magazines, on TV, or in films.

In the quest for such "perfection," many women have decided to permanently change the way they look through plastic surgery, believing such drastic measures will improve not only their features, but also their lives. One of the most popular new procedures, Botox injections, involves injecting a muscle-paralyzing substance into the upper third of the face, smoothing the skin by interrupting the nerve's signal to the injected muscle. For about six months after an injection, when the brain sends a signal down along the nerve passageway, the message doesn't reach the muscle; instead it stays motionless, causing the wrinkles to temporarily disappear. The term *botox* stands for "*bacterium Clostridium botulinum* toxin," the same illness-producing toxin found in spoiled canned goods. It's a form of botulism. In addition, a study recently published in the *Journal of Cosmetic Dermatology* reported that people who have Botox injections to get rid of lines and to make themselves look younger may in fact develop new wrinkles in different places. It seems the other muscles compensate for those temporarily unable to move in order to create facial expressions.

While I believe that medical intervention can do wonders, especially for those with severe or catastrophic disfigurements, most of us either cannot afford plastic surgery or do not want to risk its very real potential negative side effects, including temporary or permanent nerve damage, depression, skin discoloration, abnormal facial contouring, hematoma, or infection—and these are just a few of the many risks associated with several of the plastic surgery or other "beautifying" procedures.

But we have another option: makeup, which is *not* permanent! It is also a lot cheaper, carries no risks, and is at your fingertips—you don't need an expert to do it for you. And if you don't like the results, just wash your face and try again. The possibilities to create a new you are endlessly satisfying.

The women you are going to meet in this chapter are not models or beauty queens. They are, like you and me, wonderfully typical women who want to change the so-called flaws of their faces. With the quick and easy makeup techniques they learned, however, they transformed their look, becoming exceptional, striking, and hard to forget. By following several simple steps, they have learned to highlight their best features, downplay features they are uncomfortable with, and, in some cases, literally change the way their faces appear—as if by magic!

As you peruse the before and after photos, take note of the descriptions of each step. Not only will you see how easy such a transformation can be, but you will also learn how uncomplicated and straightforward these steps are for you to do on a daily basis at home!

THE COSTS OF PLASTIC SURGERY PROCEDURES FOR THE FACE

PROCEDURE	COSTS
Face-lift (including chin tuck and neck lift)	$4,000–8,000
Forehead lift	$2,400–3,200
Bleaching	$50–100 (per session; takes up to 15 sessions)
Chemical peel	$100–2,000 (depending on the area; requires several sessions)
Cheek implants	$2,000–7,500
Dermabrasion	$1,400–3,750 (requires several sessions)
Laser resurfacing	$400–2,600 (can require several sessions)
Botox injections	$175–1,000 (lasts 3–6 months)
Collagen injections	$150–1,000 (lasts 3–5 months)

The Risks of Facial Procedures

Abnormal facial contouring
Anesthesia reaction
Attached earlobe
Bleeding and blistering of the skin
Burning of the skin
Depression
Discoloration

Ear nerve damage
Facial weakness or paralysis
Hematoma
Infection
Injury to facial nerves (temporary or permanent)
Recurring fever blisters (herpes simplex)

Define Your Cheekbones and Hide That Double Chin

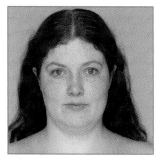

Amy wants to create definition and dimension in her face by bringing out her cheeks and hiding the hint of a double chin.

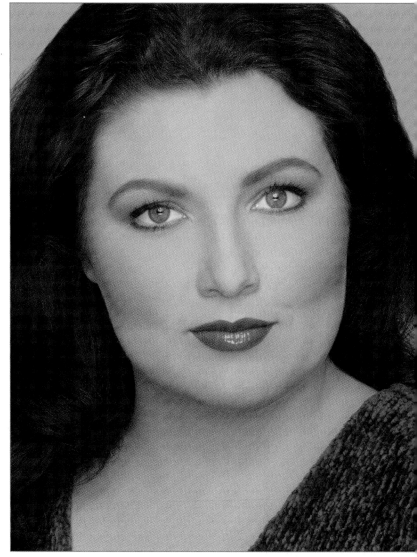

Quite a transformation! Now Amy's most prominent features seem to be her red hair, her lips, and her pretty eyes. Consider how the makeup added such dramatic contour to her face. By eliminating any trace of a double chin, and shading her cheeks and jawline using powder shadows, she dramatized her look.

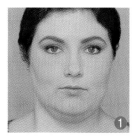

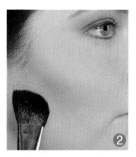

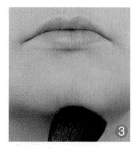

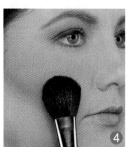

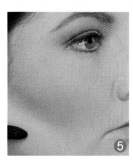

1 Apply moisturizer, light foundation, and a dusting of powder over the face.

2 Using a shader blush brush, apply a taupe shade to the hollows under the cheekbones. Any dark or earth-toned shade—taupe, burgundy, or brown—works for everyone.

3 Using the same shader blush brush, apply the taupe shadow at the base directly underneath the chin. Brush it out as far down the chin and across the jawline as needed, all the while making sure it's not too harsh.

4 Using a blush brush, apply a warm-toned blush color over the darker taupe shadow. (*Tip:* For light skin, try shades of pink or mauve, or a bronzer. For darker skin, try shades of rich brown, burgundy, pink, or orange.) Apply the blush over and above the dark contour shadow. Apply the blush starting at the top of the cheekbones, near the center of the ear, moving down toward the point of the apples of the cheeks directly under the pupils. Apply the blush over the jawline to soften the look there, as well.

5 Using a thin blender blush brush or the edge of a sponge, apply a light color underneath the dark contour shade of the cheeks. Find this color either as a blush, an eye shadow, or even a light-colored pressed powder. For light skin, try a shade that is off-white or light yellow. For dark skin, try light honey yellow, or light peach. The area you should focus on is between the cheekbone hollow and the jawline. This little trick will complete the effect in creating dimensions.

Create Contour and Add Dimension to Your Face

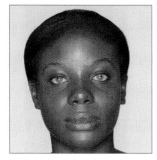

Podessa has always been very self-conscious about her blotchy, discolored skin. Before having her makeover, she was considering investing in a chemical peel or bleaching to eradicate the spots of discoloration, but was afraid of the risks of further discoloring her skin (by overbleaching), as well as the prohibitive cost. Together we worked on evening out her skin and creating more definition among her features.

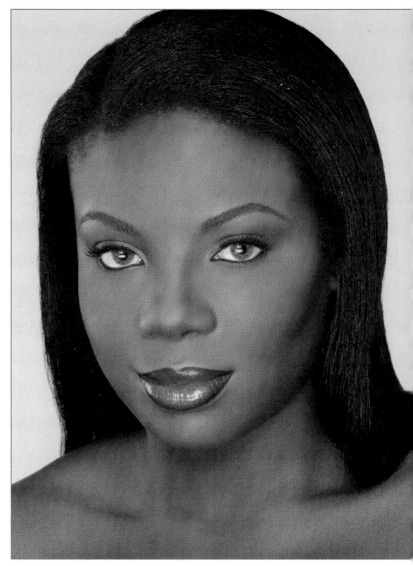

And Podessa's transformation is complete! Not only has her facial discoloration been smoothed out and eliminated, but her face also shows amazing definition compared to where she started.

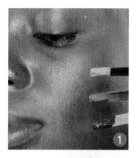

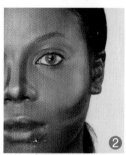

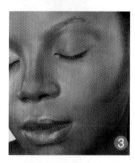

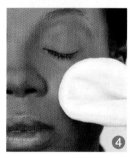

1. The interplay of three slightly different shades of foundation will help create contour and give dimension to the face. The first color should match the skin. (*Tip:* Determine your shade by testing it in the area between your cheek and jawline.) Then, for the highlights, use a color two shades lighter than the foundation base. It's best for African American women to stay in a honey tone. For the defining shade, use a color that is two shades darker than the base. (For more information on products and colors, see pages 6 and 119–120.)

2. In this photo, you see the placement for the highlighting and shading created by applying the cream foundations to the appropriate areas. Using a sponge or a brush, apply the highlight shade around the T-zone area (forehead, nose, cheekbones, and around the lips). Apply the medium skin-toned shade around the rest of the face. Using a clean concealer brush or a sponge with the dark definer shade, create hollows in the cheeks and apply around the edges of the nose to create a complementary shape for your face. Also apply the darker shade around the sides of the face (above the temples), at the hairline, and at the jawline. Contouring can be achieved with either a cream foundation or a dry powder (either a blush or an eye shadow)—it depends on what works best for you.

3. Using a sponge, smooth out the foundation. When blending, use a patting motion, gently connecting the shades together. Be careful not to eliminate the contouring that you've achieved by rubbing or blending too much.

4. Setting the foundation with powder is a crucial step in any makeup application. Use a powder puff to apply the loose powder and set the foundation in place. Try a powder that is either translucent or as light as the highlight shade, staying in a warm yellow or honey tone. Dip the powder puff into the loose powder and rub the puff's sides together to get rid of any excess powder. Pat the puff onto the face gently, using a circular motion to work the powder into the skin. (*Tip:* You can also use a brush for a more sheer application. Remember to lighly tap the brush to get rid of excess powder before using it.) Now, apply blush to the cheeks over the dark areas as well as the forehead and sides of the nose. The blush will soften any harsh dark areas.

Softening the Reds Caused by Blotches, Acne, or Rashes

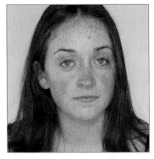

Colleen has a light complexion and a natural, soft look. Her face also features large patches of red, blotchy skin, however, which become even more visible if she gets nervous or touches her skin. This probably has an internal physical or emotional cause, stemming from either blushing or rosacea. Regardless, Colleen feels quite self-conscious and uncomfortable about her red cheeks.

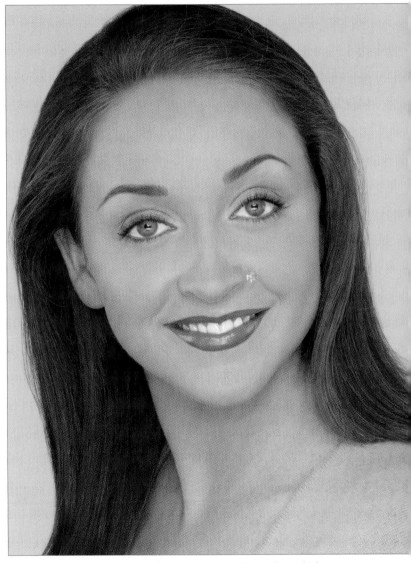

The makeup here left no trace of any redness to Colleen's skin, which now positively glows with health and vibrancy!

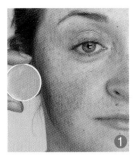

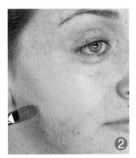

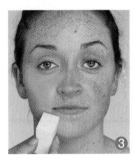

❶ With such light skin, covering the red cheeks calls for a light yellow-olive concealer cream, which should be similar to Colleen's natural skin tone but be thick enough to cover the red.

❷ Using a concealer brush, apply the concealer or foundation over any areas with redness. For smaller areas, use a smaller-tipped brush. (*Tip:* This will also work to cover red blemishes caused by hives or acne.)

❸ Using a wedge sponge, blend out the edges with a thin coat of liquid foundation. You can also gently blend the light color into the face—if so, it's not necessary to apply any foundation at all. The excess in the sponge can be used to even out the rest of the face. (Some say you should use a concealer with greenish tones—instead of yellow-olive tones—to counter the red, but when was the last time you tried to blend green with the rest of your skin tone? The light yellow-olive shade will work just fine.) Use either loose powder with a powder puff or a light dusting with a powder brush to set the cream foundation. Anytime you use a cream foundation, the best way to make sure it lasts is to set it with powder. This also prevents shades from running into each other and then eventually turning into a mushy, muddy look.

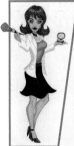

For Contouring

• Contouring means using highlights and shadows to create definition, such as by creating hollowed cheekbones, a thinner nose, or a softer jawline. There are two ways to create contour: (1) use light and dark shades of cream foundation; or (2) use dark and light shades of blush colors and eye shadows. For example, use a taupey brown to shade and a light yellow to highlight.

• Some people prefer to first apply the foundation (matching your skin tone) all over the face. Contour with the lighter highlights over the T-zone and use the dark tone to create shading elsewhere. I feel I'm saving a step by applying the three slightly different shades (light, dark, and medium) of foundation to the appropriate areas all at once.

Freckles Begone

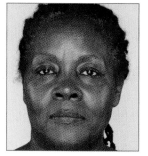

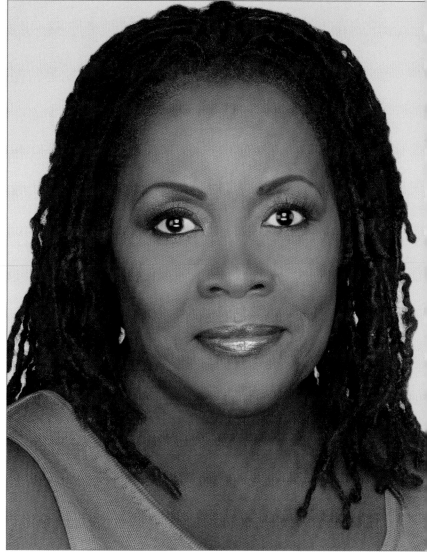

Shirley had dark, raised freckles on her face. She didn't know how to cover them up, but balked at the idea of undergoing either laser resurfacing, chemical peels or dermabrasion. As she said: "I'm not spending that kind of money!" Instead, she opted for the following makeup steps to even out her skin tone and brighten her face.

These three simple steps have completely transformed Shirley's face, giving her coverage for the freckles and a smooth, glowing complexion.

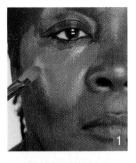

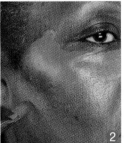

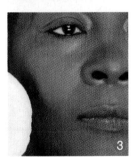

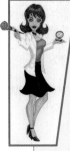

❶ Using a concealer brush and a thick concealer in a honey tone (a shade slightly lighter than Shirley's), brush over the raised freckles. The concealer shade will also be used as foundation for the T-zone (top of the forehead, nose, upper cheeks, and around the eyes and chin). Try to avoid placing the thick concealer directly under the eyes; it might get too thick and cakey. Instead, when working the foundation into the skin with a sponge, use the leftover to pat it into the delicate, sensitive area under the eyes. This will eliminate a thick clump under the eyes.

❷ Next, apply the foundation in a shade matching the skin. Remember to match the shade to the area between your jawline and the hollow of your cheek. Use either a cream or liquid foundation. Then blend the two shades together with a sponge. At the point of the colors meeting, pat gently, creating a subtle combination of shades.

❸ Using a powder puff and loose powder that is either transparent or a shade lighter than your skin color, gently set the makeup. Again, African American women should stay with honey-yellow tones: It is always easier to darken the skin with a blush or a bronzer than it is to lighten it. Once the foundation and/or setting powder gets too dark, it's quite difficult (if not impossible) to lighten it. Proceed with applying blush, eye makeup, and/or lipstick—whatever your normal routine would be.

EVE'S TIPS

For Foundation

• When applying foundation, you can choose a slightly lighter shade than your skin—especially if your complexion is oily. The oil in the skin actually turns the foundation darker over time, as it oxidizes.

• When using thick concealer as foundation, it is important to set it with powder. It will keep the foundation from running, creasing, and smudging. It will also prevent it from cracking into any lines around the eyes.

• This process will also work to cover areas with acne scars.

• The end goal when applying makeup to the face is to make the color tones of the face match your neck.

When Freckles Are Reddish

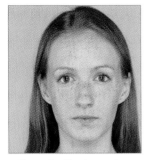

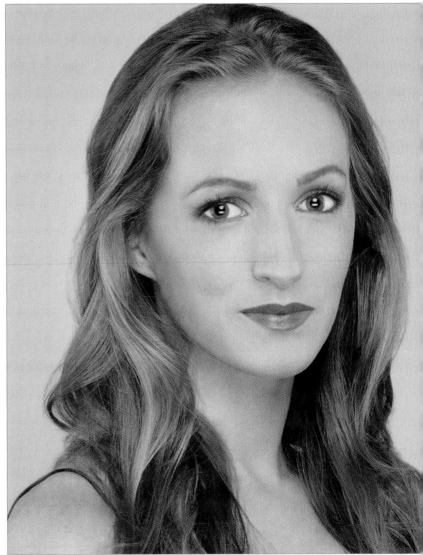

Gillian's freckles have always bothered her. She says that in the summer they are especially troublesome, since they increase in number, size, and intensity. As a young principal dancer for the American Ballet Theatre in New York City, who has to brave the spotlight often, Gillian wants her complexion to be flawless. And while some women—even those as young as Gillian—may opt for getting their skin lasered or bleached to hide the freckles, she was curious to see the magic that makeup can perform. Just take a look at her before and after shots!

As the after photo reveals, Gillian's freckles are gone, and she is thrilled.

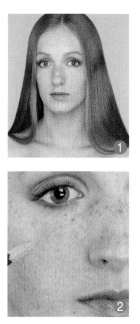

① In this photo, Gillian is wearing a sheer liquid foundation, applied with a sponge. I think she looks great, but Gillian wants to see if those freckles can be covered even further.

② Since Gillian's freckles are mostly reddish and brown and her skin is alabaster, the trick to covering the freckles is a light yellow-based cream foundation (a thicker, more opaque consistency than the sheer liquid foundation she normally wears) used over her entire face. First apply moisturizer, followed by the cream foundation applied with a sponge all over the face to cover the freckles and even out the skin tone. (*Tip:* You can also use a foundation brush to apply the cream foundation.) Don't let the thought of using a thicker cream instead of a liquid frighten you. Use it around the cheeks, forehead, and chin, and then blend the excess from the makeup sponge around the eyes and smooth out the foundation. Stay with a foundation color matching your own. Blend it gently down the neck and it will look natural.

To keep the foundation looking fresh and natural, follow with a light dusting of a neutral or light-colored loose powder using either a powder brush or a puff to set the foundation. Continue with the rest of your normal makeup routine. The key is to keep everything looking smooth.

Beauty Through the Ages

Throughout history, both women and men have altered their appearance in the name of achieving this quixotic thing called beauty.

- The Egyptians used kohl to accentuate features and trace blue veins on the skin to mimic the translucence of fair skin.
- During the Middle Ages, women wore decorative fabric patches shaped as stars, hearts, moons, or crosses on their faces to draw attention to certain features or hide scars.
- In the England of Queen Elizabeth I, it was fashionable for women to cover their faces in a thick white powder. In the queen's case, she was covering scars left by smallpox, but other women used the white powder as a sign of goodness and innocence.
- During the late eighteenth century, it was illegal in England for women to wear cosmetics. The law cited that makeup was a form of witchcraft.
- In the 1920s, it became fashionable for women to be tan. Now, at the beginning of the twenty-first century as we understand the perils of sun exposure, it is becoming more fashionable to stay out of the sun.

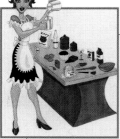

EVE'S HOME REMEDIES

- **Hair spray:** Sprayed eight inches from your face with your eyes and mouth closed, hair spray will create a sealer for your makeup.
- **Baby wipes:** These are a fast and inexpensive way to remove makeup. I use them for the celebrities on the set all the time.
- **Mud mask or wrap:** Use kitty litter (100 percent natural clay only, without additives or chemicals). Combine 1 tablespoon of clay with water to create a muddy paste. Apply to your face, letting it dry and slightly harden. Then rinse it off with warm water and a washcloth. It's easy and refreshing and will feel just like those expensive spa mud masks.
- **Cucumbers:** Crush peeled cucumbers into a pulp, and pat over your face and neck. Good for oily skin and to unclog pores.
- **Sweet almond oil** will moisturize extra-dry skin, help lashes grow, and remove makeup. It can also soothe sunburned skin.
- **Lemon juice** will dry up and help get rid of a pimple.
- **Crisco oil** will remove makeup and moisturize your skin. It can even be used to treat psoriasis and eczema.

Deemphasize Hollow Eyes

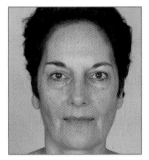

Doris is my mother-in-law. She's always had good skin along with some freckles, but she would like to alleviate the hollowness under her eyes. Like many women, Doris finds that when she applies blush to her face, it actually accentuates the hollows in that area. Instead of risking the side effects or complications of injecting fat or collagen to puff up her undereyes, however, Doris will try an easy trick to smooth out the area.

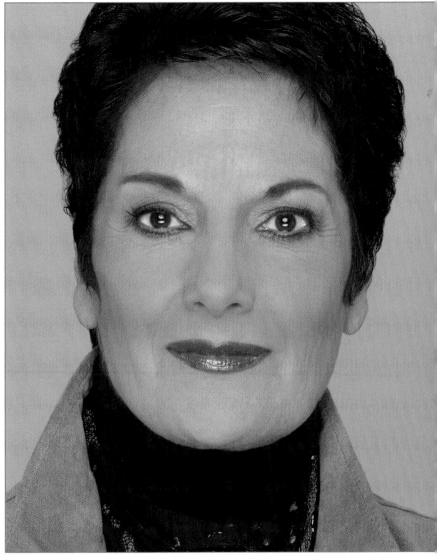

Doris is a class act all the way. She looks sexy, her skin looks moist, and the hollowness under her eyes looks much smoother.

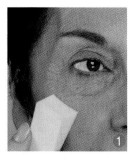

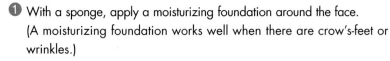 With a sponge, apply a moisturizing foundation around the face. (A moisturizing foundation works well when there are crow's-feet or wrinkles.)

② Using a concealer brush, apply a salmon-yellow concealer around the eye area and blend with the foundation. (*Tip:* Concealer can be mixed with a cream for a smoother application.)

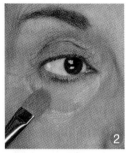

③ Using a powder puff and loose translucent powder, set the foundation.

④ Using a blush brush and a blusher shadow, apply blush starting at the top of the cheekbones, near the center of the ear, moving down toward the point on the apples of the cheeks directly under the pupils. (*Tip:* For light skin, try earth tones of mauve, pink, plum, and bronze. For darker skin, try deeper earth tones of burgundy, bronze, pink, and orange.) For added effect, smile and place shadow blush on the apples of the cheeks. When applying a cream blush, smile, dab the cream on the apples of the cheeks, and blend it back toward the center of the ear.

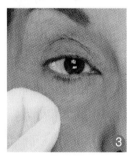

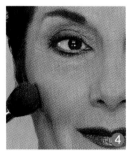

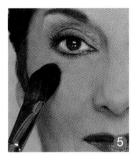

⑤ Using a thin blender blush brush, apply a neutral or light powder (two or three shades lighter than the blush) at the edges of the blush on the cheeks, blending it out. Continue applying the lighter shade on the hollow under the eye. Remember, blending is the key to having your makeup look flawless.

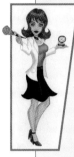

For Blush

• The purpose of blush is to give a healthy glow and help in creating the dimension of contours to the face. Using the light and dark shades properly is the key to creating dimension.

• If you've applied too much blush and it looks a bit too harsh or clownlike, smooth it out by blending away the edges with a neutral or light powder at the edges of the blush. You can also just wipe away the excess by gently dabbing a clean makeup sponge or puff across the area.

• Avoid placing very light shades (off-white or yellow) directly over very dark shades. When they mix together, it can look like a patch of grayish dirt. Keep the very light shade about a quarter inch below the very dark shade.

• Using a blush brush, apply blush starting at the top of the cheekbones, near the center of the ear, moving down toward the point on the apples of the cheeks directly under the pupils.

• When shading, use a color two to three shades darker than your own skin tone.

• To locate the bottom cheekbone hollows, suck in your cheeks. The area that does not have a bone is the hollow.

• When applying the darker blush shadow, use the thin part of the brush and begin at the edge of the cheek next to the ear. Using very little of the dark blush shadow color, begin at the edge near the ear and work your way out to where the cheekbone ends (not reaching the area under the pupil). If you're not sure of where the cheekbone ends, it's safer to keep the shading short rather than extending it out too far and having it look like a patch of dirt.

Bye-Bye Crow's-Feet and Laugh Lines

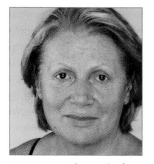

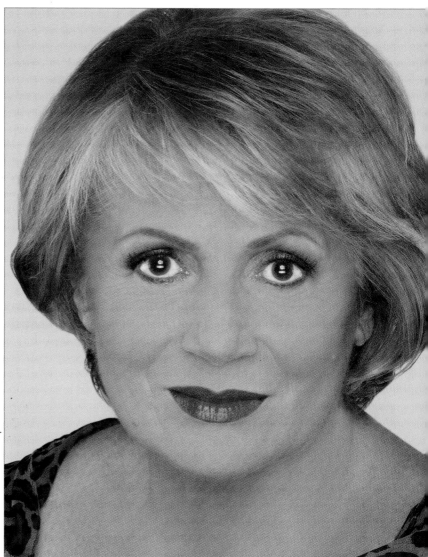

Riva is my mother and, of course, I think she is perfectly beautiful. She, too, works in the theater industry, and like many women of her gentle age, she has become almost obsessed with the crow's-feet around her eyes and lips. She also didn't like the lines on her forehead and the deep laugh lines on her cheeks. And though Riva has considered having surgery "to get rid of everything," she's afraid—of both the pain and the results. In her line of work, Riva has seen too many people lose all the character and personality of their face after cosmetic surgery. It didn't take much convincing to show her that makeup was an easier answer to her worries.

As you can see in Riva's after photo, the lines that were driving her crazy are dramatically deemphasized. The makeup highlights her eyes and lips, even giving her cheekbones more elegant prominence. She now looks like a beautiful woman aging gracefully—without the use of a scalpel or a laser!

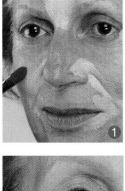

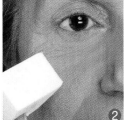

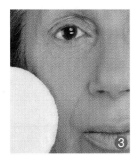

1 Using a concealer brush, apply a concealer or highlighter in a shade slightly lighter than your foundation color to the areas that might be a bit sunken in. For light skin, try highlighting with tones of very light peach, very light ivory, or very light yellow. If you have darker skin, try highlighting with light peach-honey tones, or light yellow-honey tones. Highlighting around the laugh lines, the edges of the eyes, and the forehead and lip areas will bring them out and give the illusion of being less sunken in. If the concealer or highlighter feels too thick, mix it with some moisturizer or the foundation. Think of it as the two-step process of spackling and painting: You fill in the holes and crevices before applying the next and final layer, which is foundation, as you'll see below. You can also use your finger to apply the concealer. The heat in your finger will melt the concealer into the crevices.

2 Using a makeup sponge, apply your foundation, which matches the skin (check on the side of the face, between the jawline and the hollow of the cheek). When going over and blending with the highlighted areas, be careful not to rub off all the highlights. Pat the foundation on top of the highlight and gently blend the two together. Remember, there are no set rules for applying makeup, and in this situation you have the option of first applying foundation and then highlighting the areas you need to. It's up to you and what you feel works best for you.

3 With a powder puff, use translucent loose powder to set the foundation. Continue with the rest of the makeup application as you would normally.

Instant Face-Lift
(No Pain, Absolute Gain)

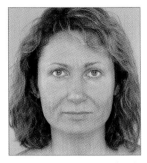

How could I subject my family and friends to being photographed as their most vulnerable premakeup selves and let their features be displayed for all to see, without including myself in the mix? So here I am, front and center. As many women tend to do to themselves, I, too, can look at myself and focus on my imperfect features. I notice my acne scars (caused by teenage cystic acne, which left red blotches on my pale skin). I also notice my uneven eyes, which have begun their inevitable drooping process; my nose, which could be thinner; my laugh lines and uneven lips, which I would like to hide.

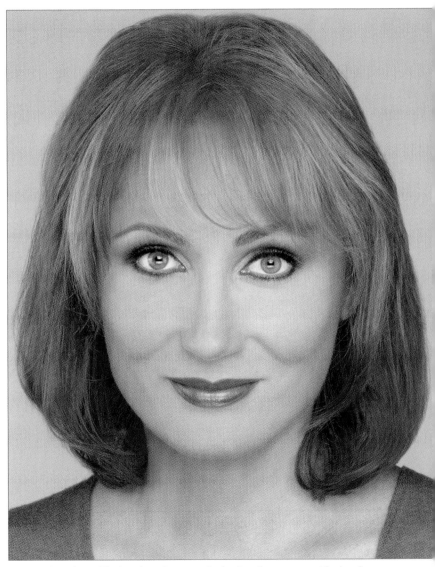

My eyes have been lifted and my face stretched, all without surgery. The laugh lines and acne scars are not as deep; my eyes appear to be more open and awake. Talk about a miracle cure!

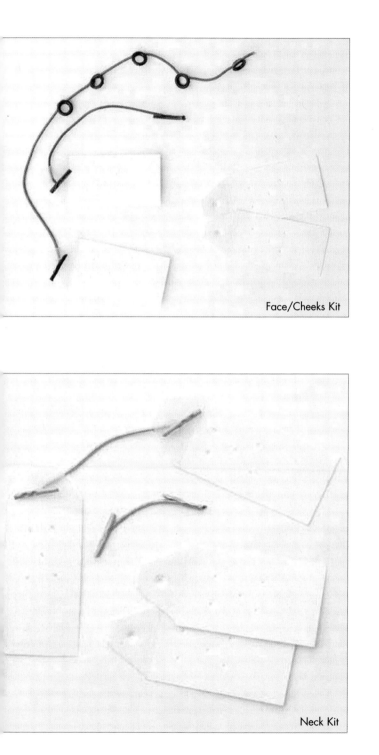

Face/Cheeks Kit

Neck Kit

Imagine all that plastic surgery I could indulge in—yet not only would it cost a fortune, but also I'm too frightened of the pain and risk! Take a look at the magical cure that follows.

You'll begin by using a face-lift kit (found in specialty makeup supply stores). These pieces are available in several sizes to fit the face and neck. There are separate sets for the eyes, the cheeks and face, and the neck. Here I am using the sets for the eyes and the cheeks and face.

Each process involves a set of two elastic pieces, one long and the other short; one side has an attachment for an individual piece of tape, while the other is able to combine with and hook into the first. The tape is placed on the face. The elastic will run through and be hidden by the hair. The two elastic pieces meet behind the head and connect. (Several loops and hooks allow the pieces to adjust to any size face.) Once connected, any excess elastic remaining in the back can be cut off. When the set is hooked together, a bobby pin will help keep it in place. (This is kept underneath and hidden by the hair.) The kits come with spare tapes to use and cut to size.

Separate sections in the hair running horizontally across the back of the head create a smooth path for the elastic pieces.

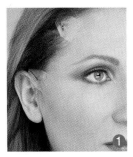

1 After applying regular makeup, place the short-sided elastic tape above your temples. Place the long-sided elastic tape on the other side of your face, above the temples as well. Run the elastic across the hair to the back and connect the two elastic pieces. Cut any excess elastic. This will pull up the eyes and create an eye-lift effect.

Follow the same process with the tapes, this time placing the short piece just above the ear, with the long elastic piece on the other side. Run through the back and connect the two pieces. Cut off any excess elastic. This will pull up the cheeks, creating a face-lift effect.

2 Using a concealer brush, apply concealer or foundation over the shiny tape pieces and powder to set. Pull down the hair to cover all traces of the tapes and elastic. Note that face-lift tapes can be applied before or after your makeup.

Tools for Your Face

These are the tools used on the ladies for their makeovers:

- Moisturizer
- Sponge
- Powder puff
- Brushes: concealer, powder, blush
- Concealers: a variety of shades to highlight, contour, and enhance
- Foundation: a variety of textures and shades
- Loose powders: neutral and darker
- Blush shadows: a variety of shades
- Face-and-cheek-, eye-, or neck-lift kits

As you've seen, not all the women used all of these products or tools. Once you understand your own needs, you will be able to select the tools that will be most effective for your particular face. In chapter 7, More About the Tools of the Trade, you will learn more specific information about the tools, what they are used for, and how to select them.

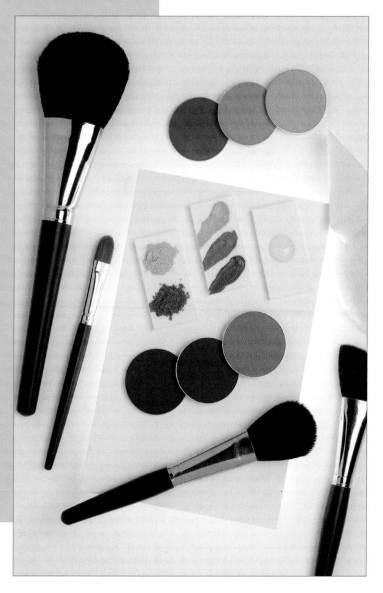

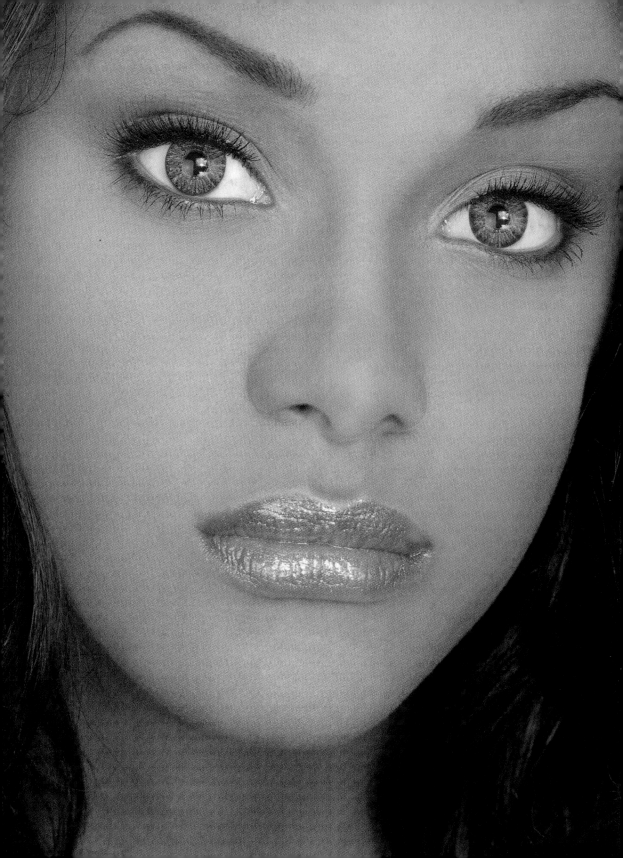

CHAPTER

3

the eyes

&

the brows

HOW TO OPEN THE WINDOWS
OF YOUR FACE

O! What a life is the eye!
What a strange and inscrutable essence!
Samuel Taylor Coleridge

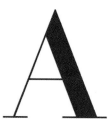sapphire-blue night sky, the new spring's green, a golden-crimson sunrise that gently unfolds the dawn of a new day before you—we witness these majesties of nature through our eyes. Indeed, it is through our eyes that we first know the world around us. And it's through our eyes that we first communicate with the world. As the most expressive part of our face, our eyes can reveal our most complicated emotions, gaze out in love, or connect with others at the level of the unspoken.

Capable of such power, then, it is no wonder that throughout history each generation has focused on enhancing and opening up the eyes, making them more dramatic and appealing. And yet how we have approached this task has changed along the way. Just as many of us may long for fuller lips, more defined cheekbones, or smaller noses, we also want to make adjustments to our eyes and eyebrows. Is plastic surgery necessary? Of course not. Yet many women still feel they need to turn to surgeons and their knives in order to combat the effects of aging and give their eyes more shape and vibrancy. I say, try makeup first—you have nothing to lose and everything to gain!

Using several simple makeup techniques, you can learn how to enhance and accentuate your own miraculous eyes and literally change the nature of your face. Five of the women in this chapter highlight the most common issues concerning women about their eyes: dark circles, definition, opening up, and lifting. But before we get to the eyes themselves, we need to address the eyebrows. Most women find that once they trim, sculpt, or hone their eyebrows, they are able to see their eyes (and the issues they want to address) in a whole new way. When you shape your eyebrows, you necessarily open up and clear the way for further enhancing the natural beauty of your eyes. Let's take a look at the startling transformations that follow, and how the women followed simple steps to achieve such dramatic results.

The Five Most Popular Eye Procedures

- Eye lift
- Eyelid surgery
- Correction of crow's-feet
- Bleaching of dark circles
- Correction of heavy lids and bags under the eyes

The costs for the various eye procedures range between $1,800 and $3,500, depending on how many individual treatments are performed. The risks are extensive, including infection, nerve damage, reaction to anesthesia, and hematomas. Because the skin around the eyes is so delicate and sensitive, these procedures often need to be repeated with time.

Eyebrows

Just as we like to open and accentuate the shape of our eyes, so, too, we like to shape our eyebrows. Even more than eye makeup, the shapes of eyebrows vary from fashion trend to fashion trend. In the theater, a change of eyebrows can define a character—from an evil queen to an innocent young maiden, from a Kabuki performer to a court jester, from a fairy princess to a monster. The shape of the eyebrows sets the tone for the rest of the face.

Brow trends change constantly. In the 1930s and 1940s, women tended to imitate Hollywood's leading ladies, plucking their brows into the same slim crescents worn by Bette Davis, Marlene Dietrich, and Mae West. The 1950s saw boldly shaped brows popularized by Sophia Loren, Elizabeth Taylor, Ingrid Bergman, Audrey Hepburn, and Marilyn Monroe. During the 1970s, Brooke Shields and other natural beauties barely touched their brows, letting them grow into bushy fullness. Fortunately, you don't need to go to extremes; you can be in fashion by simply working with what you've got. From thin and arched to bushy and everything in between, you, too, can learn how best to tweeze, wax, pluck, shave, thread, bleach, or cut your brows in the way you wish.

While I believe there is no one way to treat eyebrows, I do think there is a best way to approach your eyebrows: First, decide what kind of look you are after, and then decide what kind of brow shape best complements your eye shape, face, and overall look.

The Subtle Arch

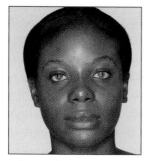

When we began our makeover session, Podessa told me that she wanted to achieve a softer, more elegant appearance. Although you can see that Podessa's eyebrows have a beautiful natural arch to them, they could be shaped a bit more so that they echo the contour of her eyes more discreetly.

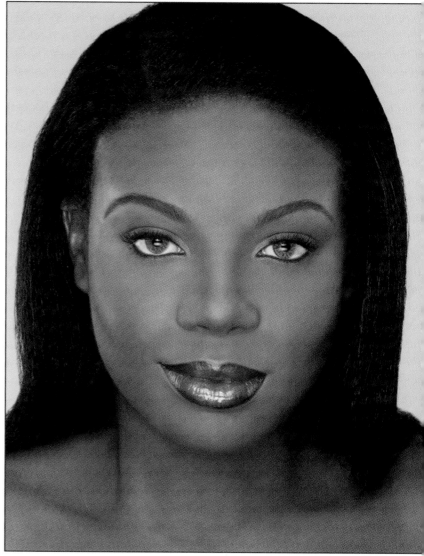

As you can see, following trimming and plucking, Podessa's eyebrows now echo the natural arch of her eyes, further dramatizing her exotic look.

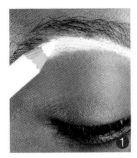

1. With a white pencil, outline the area you want to pluck. The white line will help you see if you like the shape that you intend to keep. Remember, if your hair is very light, you can darken the area you want to keep using a dark brown pencil.

2. Using a good gripping pair of tweezers, grasp individual hairs near their roots. With swift, sharp movements, pluck the hair in the white area in the direction it's growing. Try to remove one row at a time. (*Tip:* You can also use a razor to shave the hairs drawn in white.)

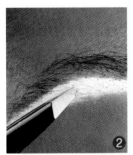

3. With a spooly, which looks like a clean mascara brush, brush up and hold down the brow hairs. Using small scissors (those used for cutting cuticles or baby nails), trim the excess brow hairs. Try not to cut too much hair off.

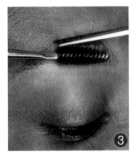

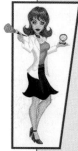

Shaping Your Eyebrows

- The eyebrow should begin directly above the inner corner of your eye. To find the highest point of the arch, hold a pencil parallel to the outside edge of the iris. The first three-quarters of the brows should head upward toward your natural peak; the final quarter should head downward and taper off at the end. From the arch to the outer corner of the eye, your brow should fall in a straight or slightly curved line, depending on the look you're trying to achieve.
- To determine brow length, hold a pencil from your nostril to the outside edge of your eye. The point at which the pencil touches your brow is your perfect brow length.
- To create the perfect arch at home, you should first mark the area accurately. Remember, if your eyebrows are very light, then fill in what you want to keep with a dark color. If your brows are unruly, use brow gel to keep them in place.
- Use a moisturizer or makeup remover to clean off any remaining white color from the pencil left on the brows.
- Use an astringent to disinfect and clean the plucked area.
- Filling in the brows: Brush the brows downward with a spooly. Use a pencil to draw a line along the upper edge of the brow to define the arch. Comb the brows upward and outward.
- Fill in sparse areas with a freshly sharpened brow pencil. Use light, quick feathering strokes to draw in the hair. Brow powder will give the brows overall definition and a more natural look.

Debunking an Eyebrow Myth

You may have heard the myth that you should never pluck above the eyebrow. In fact, to create the perfect arch, you might need to eliminate unwanted hair above your eyebrow. It's fine to do so. We pluck and eliminate hair all over our face. Who made up the rule that we should never pluck above the eyebrow? Unwanted hair grows below and above the brows.

To Pluck Above the Brows or Not?

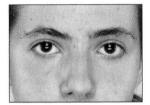

Tamara is my niece and a teenager. Like many girls her age, she needs to care for her eyebrows. In the past, Tamara used to get her eyebrows waxed or plucked, both of which caused her pain and always made her fear getting them done again. For Tamara, I actually used the same outlining technique as with Podessa and then removed the unwanted hair with a brow razor. It was quick and painless. Tamara now can just maintain the shape using the same brow razor. (The brow razor is not as sharp as a standard razor. It's also quite safe and easy to use.) No pain, with all the gain. I was able to delicately shave below and above Tamara's brows to create the appropriate shape for her.

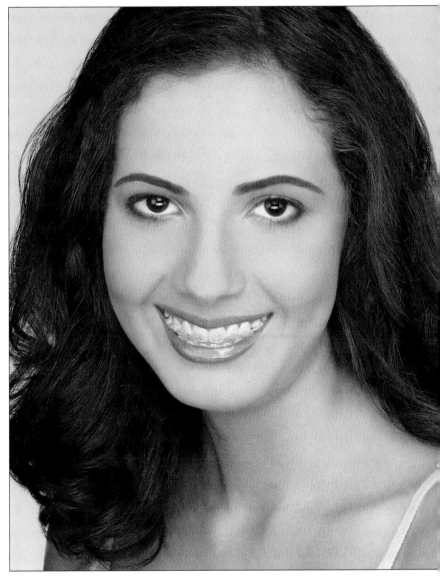

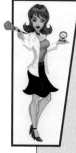

For the Brows

- Try using a hair conditioner on your brows when shaping them with a razor. It will soften the brows for easier shaving, condition them, and lay them flat for better control.
- Avoid getting creative with your waxing the day before an important event.
- The best time to tweeze brows is after a shower or bath, when your hair is at its most pliable; this will make for easier and less painful plucking.
- Avoid overtweezing your eyebrows.
- To slightly lighten the eyebrows and soften your look, try a cream bleach. Leave it on for five to fifteen minutes, depending on your original shade and skin sensitivity.
- For the most natural results when filling in and shaping eyebrows, use a brow pencil, brow powder, cream brow color, or brow mascara. Select a color the same shade or a shade lighter than your own eyebrows.
- Fill in the eyebrows with a shade one or two tones lighter than your own if you have dark hair. (If your brows are very light, try a shade one or two tones darker.)
- Try to stay in shades of warm browns or taupes. These look more natural and soften the appearance.
- Avoid using black to fill in the eyebrows. It can have a tendency to appear a bit harsh and might turn grayish.
- If you've overcolored your eyebrows or made them too dark, use a hard toothbrush dipped in a neutral powder or shadow and lightly brush over the brows.
- Eyebrow shapes are a very personal choice. My advice would be to stay away from fads and stick with the most flattering look for your face. Avoid overplucking, since the hairs don't always grow back. Try to follow your own eyebrows' natural shape. But if you're not sure, go to a professional the first time you have your brows plucked, and let the expert shape your brows. Then you will be able to maintain the shape yourself.

Tools for Your Brows

- Pencils
- Powder shadow
- Scissors
- Spooly brush
- Tweezers
- Eyebrow brush

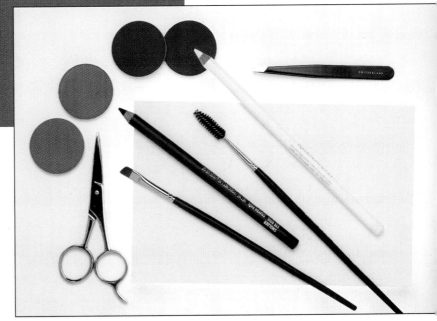

The Eyes

Now you are ready to consider your eyes. As you learned above, your eyebrows add essential balance to your face, bringing together all your features into a harmonious whole. But the eyes are the real focus of your face. Many women are concerned about dark circles under their eyes—caused by either genetics, poor circulation, alcohol, or toxins—and the bluish tint of the underlying blood vessels. Some want their eyes "lifted," their crow's-feet removed, or more defined creases in their eyelids. Whatever feature you want to accentuate or deaccentuate, let's see how the following women have opened their faces and made room for their wondrous eyes.

Get Rid of Dark Circles and Lift the Eyes

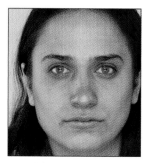

Rachel felt that her eyebrows were unruly and needed sculpting. But she was also concerned about the dark circles around her eyes, and wanted to "lift" her lids so that her eyes appeared bigger. Such dark pigmentation in this area is hereditary for many women, even though people often assume that lack of sleep is the problem. Instead of lightening her circles with laser or a bleaching product or lifting her eyes surgically, Rachel decided to try out these simple steps.

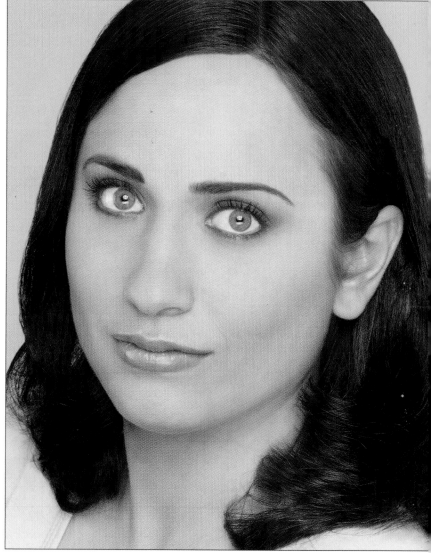

Take a look at how magically a few delicate touches in the right places hide those dark circles and open up Rachel's face, allowing her eyes to embolden it. Her eyes are more open and bright, all while still maintaining a natural look.

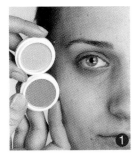

❶ To cover up the dark blue-purple-red circles under the eyes, use a salmon or light peach concealer. The exact shade of salmon or light peach will vary, depending on the hue of your skin. Avoid using a concealer that's light yellow, whitish, or anything in that color family (such as the top concealer in photo): It can turn the dark blue circles grayish and create raccoon eyes. Most brands offer a salmon or light peach shade; the color is closer to that of a cheese doodle than a potato chip!

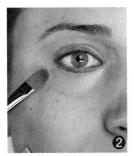

❷ Using a concealer brush, apply concealer to the dark area beneath and above the eyelid. (*Tip:* You can also use your finger. The heat in the finger will help blend the concealer into the face.) If the concealer is too thick or dry, mix it with a moisturizer or with the foundation.

    Apply foundation as needed around the face—use as little or as much as you are comfortable with. Here we used a light application of a liquid yellow-based foundation because Rachel's face has red pigmentation, and yellow works best to cover up reddish tones.

    Then, using a powder brush, dust with loose powder to set over the face. Apply the powder with a sponge or wedge underneath and above the eyelid to set the concealer.

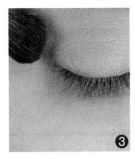

❸ Using an allover eye brush, apply a light neutral eye shadow over the entire eyelid. (*Tip:* The lighter and larger you make your lid, the larger and more open the eye will appear to be.)

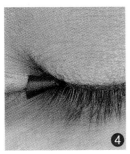

❹ Using a brown or taupe pencil, line all over the top of the lash line. Line the bottom lash line only from the edge to halfway inward. This will elongate the eye, yet still keep it looking natural.

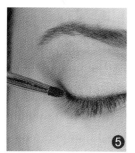

⑤ With a smudger brush and a dark eye shadow, smudge out the pencil lines by going over the area with the liner. Use short up-and-down strokes and stay close to the edge of the lash line, creating a softer line and smoking the lashes out.

⑥ Using a blender brush, apply a medium warm earth-toned eye shadow in the crease of the eye with a back-and-forth motion about three or four times. Using the crease opens up the eye by allowing you to make the lid as large as possible. The dark crease will draw attention to wherever it's placed, giving the effect of a more open eye.

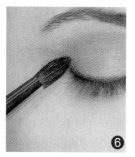

⑦ Using a definer brush, apply the same dark eye shadow to define the crease area, giving dimension to the eye. Avoid using too much shadow here; keep the dark crease thin and subtle. Creating or defining a crease area allows you to open up the eye.

⑧ With the same allover brush, use the same light neutral color that you applied to the lid to blend and smooth out the browbone area. (This is basically a cleanup step in case you overextended the eye shadow.) Try to keep this area looking light and clean.

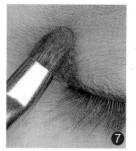

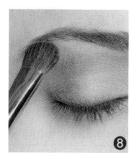

"Smoke Out" Your Eyes

To "smoke out" means to use a dark shadow and create a soft effect. It will hold the liner and keep it from smudging, creasing, or coming off. It will also give you the ability to extend, elongate, and enlarge the shape of the eye with a soft shadow. For example, when an eye shadow is applied over a harsh liquid liner, you can still achieve a softer effect by bringing out the eye.

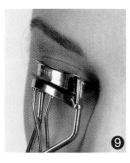

9 One of the last steps is curling your lashes, to give them that seductive movie-star look. Curling your lashes makes them appear thicker—translation, *sexier*. The key here is to get the lash curler as close to the lash line as possible. As you close the curler, push it upward toward the eyelid—this is what actually curls the lashes. Work it out gently, curling two or three times as you pull it outward to the end of the lashes, squeezing as you go. This will look like a natural curl rather than a dent in the lashes.

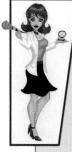

10 Apply mascara as soon as you curl the lashes. If you apply several coats and they clump together, just use a lash separator—but carefully!

EVE'S TIPS

For Eyelashes

- If you're using a metal curler, try using a hair dryer to heat the curler's center. Like a curling iron, it will hold the curl longer. Just be careful not to overheat it, because that can be painful.
- For those of us who are a bit clumsy when it comes to curling and applying mascara, it's best to do both before beginning the eye makeup application. This way, whatever you smudge, just clean off; you don't need to ruin your eye makeup. Do whatever feels comfortable for you. I usually curl and apply mascara before beginning my own makeup. Some people smudge their mascara all over the lid when applying. This can ruin a nice makeup job.

Larger, More Defined Eyes

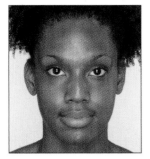

Tiffany has a natural, fresh look, but she would like to lighten up her face and bring out the natural almond shape of her eyes.

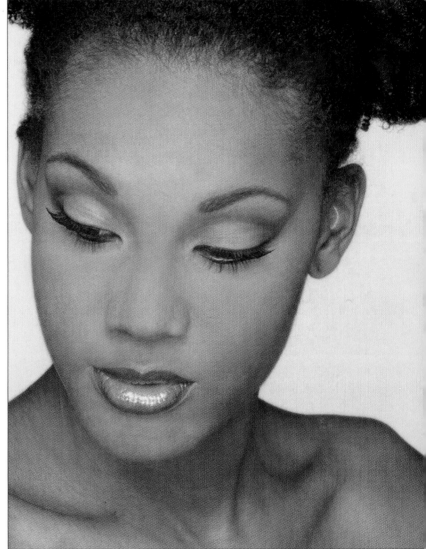

Tiffany's makeup brings together three arresting features of her face: her beautiful wide-set eyes, her fully arched brows, and her strong jawline. Her face, which has always been open and inviting, is now even more so with the added touch of makeup.

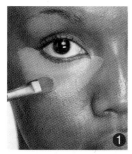

1 Using a concealer brush, apply a honey-toned concealer lighter than the skin shade. Avoid overly yellow or olive hues, because they have a tendency to turn ashy. It's best to use shades lighter than your own complexion to cover the T-zone (the area across your forehead, down and around the nose to your chin) and around the eye area.

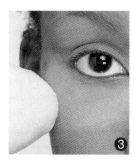

2 With a sponge, apply foundation (liquid or cream) to the rest of the face. Tiffany's face, like those of some other African American women, is darker than the rest of her body, neck, and chest, so a lighter foundation than her face is used. The object is for the face to match the neck and the rest of the body; we've all seen women whose face is a different shade from their neck and rest of the body—it looks like they went to a tanning parlor from the neck up!

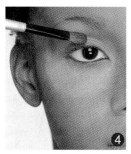

3 Using a powder puff, apply loose powder to set the foundation. With the powder, like the foundation, stay with a lighter shade. (You can always make it darker; it's easier to darken than it is to lighten up.)

4 With an allover eye shadow brush, use a light-honey-toned, neutral eye shadow over the entire lid area. (*Tip:* You can apply extra loose powder under the eye area to catch excess eye shadow that might fall there. When you're done with the eye makeup, just dust off the loose powder and any shadow that has fallen.)

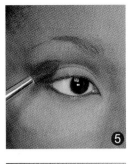

⑤ Using a blender brush, apply a medium-toned eye shadow to outline the crease area with a back-and-forth motion. Try to extend the crease area toward the outer corner of the eye. This will elongate and create a larger-looking eye with a sexy shape.

⑥ Using an eyeliner brush, apply liquid black liner as close to the lash line as possible. (*Tip:* When applying liquid liner, to prevent a big smudge at the inner corner of your eye, begin at the center and work your way out. Then, with the excess left on the brush, go to the inner corner and complete the line.) At the outer edge, angle the liner slightly and move up and out, then line the bottom of the lash line with a black pencil. For added effect, you can also draw inside the lash line area.

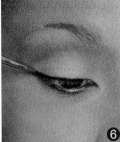

⑦ Using a definer brush, apply a dark shadow over the liner to smudge and smoke it out. Then extend the outer eye and define the crease area, keeping the dark shading thin and subtle.

⑧ Using the same allover brush, apply the light eye shadow used for the lid on the browbone. This step is to smooth out the darker shadows and highlight the browbone.

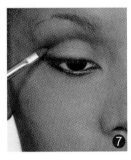

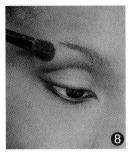

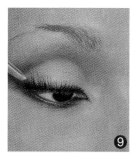

9 If you want to add false lashes for more dramatic effect, measure the lashes onto your own and then cut off the ends of the false lashes to size. You're better off making them too short than too long; if the lashes are too lengthy, they will seem to close the eyes rather than open them up—the very opposite of what you are attempting to achieve. Using tweezers to hold them up, apply glue to the lashes and place them as close to the lash line as possible. (See Accentuate the Eyes, later in this chapter, for more detailed directions for application of false eyelashes.)

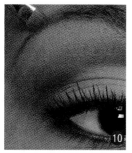

10 Fill in the brows with a shade lighter than your own. I prefer a brown or reddish shade here.

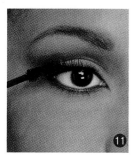

11 Apply mascara while looking down. And remember to avoid pumping the brush into the applicator too many times during each application; this only lets air into the tube and dries out the mascara faster.

A More Defined Eyelid Crease

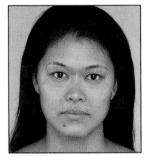

Like many Asian Americans, Sung Yun has considered eye surgery to remove the top layer of her skin, a procedure that would remove the fold over the eye in order to create a lid and bring out the eyes. Such a procedure is costly and permanent, however, and Sung Yun has had the foresight to know that there may come a day when she better appreciates the natural almond shape of her eyes. Here is a way for Sung Yun to create more definition in her eyelids without the permanency.

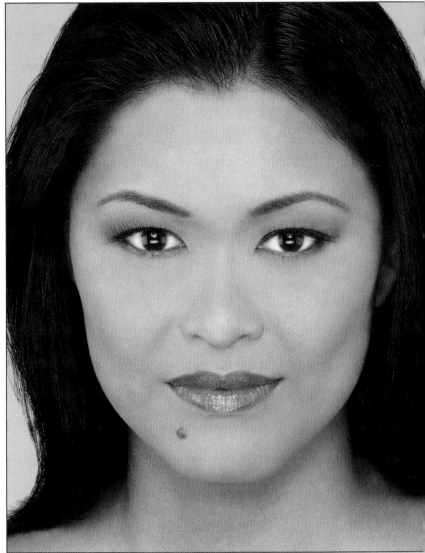

With just a few magical brush strokes, Sung Yun artfully added dimension to her beautiful almond-shaped eyes.

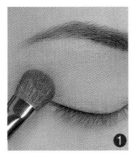

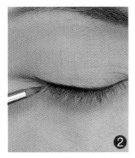

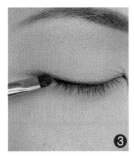

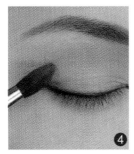

❶ Apply a light moisturizer and base as usual. Using an eye shadow brush, apply a light neutral eye shadow over the entire lid.

❷ Using an eyeliner brush, apply either a cream or a liquid liner to the lash line. (*Tip:* When applying liner, begin by placing the brush as close to the lash line as possible in the middle of the eye. Then, with the leftover liner on the brush, go to the inner edge of the eye. This way, you avoid creating a smudge at the inner edge of your eye with too much liner.) It does not need to be a perfect line; just try to get it as close to the lash as possible and extend it out and up at the outside edge of the eye.

❸ Apply a smudger brush dipped in a dark eye shadow (brown, purple, blue, black) over the line to blend and smoke it out. This way, you can go over and cover up any mistakes made drawing the line while softening the effect of the liner.

❹ Using a blender brush and a medium-warm eye shadow (brown, purple, pink, orange, mauve), apply to the center of the eyelid area, using back-and-forth (windshield-wiper-like) strokes that create a mild crease in the desired area.

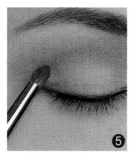

⑤ Using a definer brush and a dark eye shadow (this can be the same dark shade that you used to smoke out the liner), define the area to appear like the crease. (Try to keep it thin.) If it comes out too dark or thick, just repeat the medium shade and blend again. Remember, blending is key to makeup looking flawless and natural.

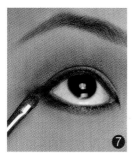

⑥ Use a pencil (black, brown, purple) to line the bottom of the lash line, staying as close to the lash line as possible. Lining the bottom of the lash line is a matter of choice: A line can be drawn all over the bottom, from the center outward, or not at all. A line all over will give a dramatic effect. An even more dramatic look is to line with a dark color inside the eyelash area both on the bottom and on top— but be cautious with this one. A line from the center outward will extend the eye out and create a more natural look. No line at all will keep the focus on the upper part of the eye.

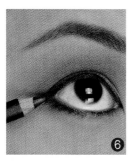

⑦ Using the smudger brush, apply the dark eye shadow over the line to soften the look and smoke it out. When reaching the connecting edges of the top and bottom liners, extend the shadow at the outer corners. This will make the eye appear larger.

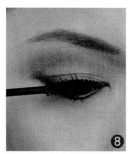

⑧ After curling the lashes, apply mascara. Sometimes we get a bit messy with mascara. If you prefer, you can curl and mascara your lashes before beginning any of the shadow steps. This way, if you get smudges, they are easily cleaned up without ruining the eye shadow.

Fill in the brows with a loose powder (one to two shades lighter). Brownish tones are good, but try to avoid using black to fill in the brows. Black has a tendency to look a bit harsh and might sometimes look gray. The lighter color will still fill in and look softer.

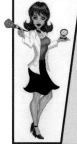

For the Eyes

- A white pencil can be applied to the inner lash line of the eye. This can create the effect of a larger eye. Still, it can also have a tendency to look like you're trying too hard.

- Placing a light shimmer under the bottom eyeliner will soften and give added oomph to the eye.

- I prefer using black mascara to achieve the most dramatic effect. I apply only one coat and it does the trick. Brown mascara works better if you want a more natural look; it's also a good option if you are very fair-skinned or a young adult.

- When using eyeliners, I prefer using shades of black and brown. To add extra color, you can always smoke out the effect with a blue, green, wine, or other eye shadow. Using color in this way still achieves the effect of a liner, and, with added shimmer, gives a softer look.

- For basic eye colors—whether in pencils or shadows—I prefer using neutral tones. Try ivory, beige, taupe, mauve, brown, bronze, wine, or gray, and try varying in the depth and intensity of each. Color can always be added to small areas to give that extra effect.

- The "blue" myth. Some tell you never to wear blue if you have blue eyes; others say never wear blue at all. I say, if you like blue, go ahead and wear it. Apply it as an accent color over a neutral; it will blend in quite nicely without screaming, I'm wearing blue!

Make Older Eyes
Look Young Again

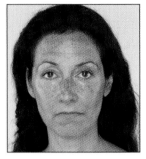

Claudia would like to brighten up her eyes and make them come alive. So we set out to eliminate the slight signs of aging by addressing the extra folds developing above her eyes, as well as the area around her eyes, where crow's-feet have appeared. Claudia is also looking for a way to eliminate the dark bluish, almost purple, tone underneath her eyes as well as bring out the luster in her green eyes.

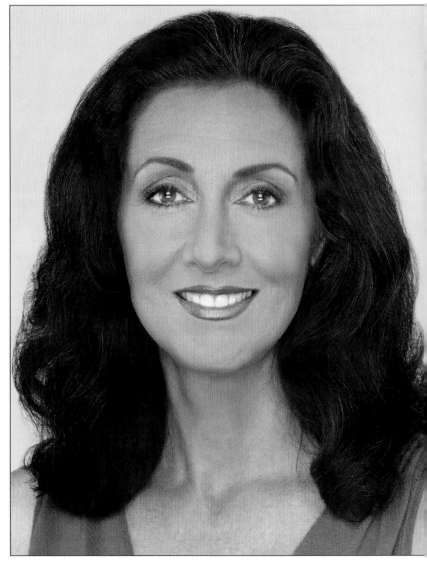

In this after shot of Claudia, you have a good view of the subtle layering of colors and contours that heighten her eyes so dramatically, taking away any distracting effects of her crow's-feet.

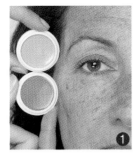

❶ Mix a salmon or light peach concealer (such as the bottom concealer in photo) with a moisturizer and apply it with a concealer brush to blend it into the foundation (liquid or cream).

❷ When there are lines and crow's-feet under the eyes, powder with a motion going inward toward the nose. I prefer using a sponge in the delicate eye area, while gently patting in the powder. Think of it as going into the grooves. The powder will actually keep the foundation from moving and caking up into the lines.

❸ With a large eye shadow brush, apply a light or medium-warm shadow (shiny) on the lid. The shiny lid will look dewy, healthy, and youthful.

❹ With a blender brush, apply a medium-warm eye shadow, adding curvy back-and-forth strokes to the crease about three or four times. Then, from the outer edge of the crease, go backward, staying at the lash line up to the center of the eye.

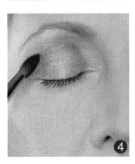

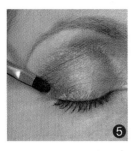

⑤ Using a definer brush with a darker eye shadow, define the crease and edge of the eyelid. Try to keep the dark shade minimal and thin—it's there to define the crease and create dimension.

⑥ Use a dark creamy pencil (brown, black, blue, purple) on the top and bottom of the lash line. A liquid liner can also be used on the top lash line.

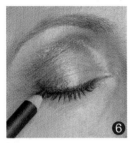

⑦ With a smudger brush, apply the same dark eye shadow that you used to define the crease over the eyeliner. This will soften and smoke out the pencil line; it will also blend out any mistakes or hard edges on both the top and bottom of the lash line and keep the pencil line in place.

⑧ Using an eyebrow brush and a light taupey eye shadow, fill in and define the eyebrows.

⑨ Curl the lashes and apply mascara to complete the look.

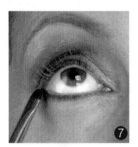

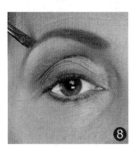

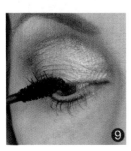

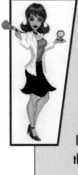

EVE'S TIPS

Ordinarily, people want to cover up dark blue or purple with a yellow concealer. Unfortunately, all that will do is create a green or grayish color and make Claudia look more like a raccoon, only accentuating the darkness rather than camouflaging it. The shade to use to cover up blue or purple under the eye is a salmon or light peach color to neutralize the bluish tone and match the skin.

Accentuate the Eyes to Downplay Other Features

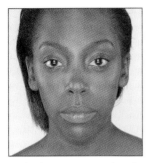

Kimberly is a petite rock-and-roll singer with a tiny, delicate face. Without resorting to eye surgery or bleaching, she wants to deemphasize the pigmentation under her eyes and shift attention away from her chin toward her eyes. There are a few steps we can take to accentuate her eyes and bring her many lovely features into more focus.

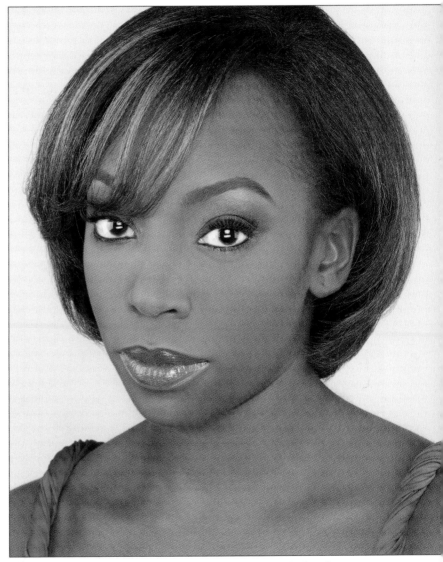

Kimberly used the makeup not only to cover her undereye circles but also to create a smoky look around her eyes. She has made the most of the dramatic space between her eyes and brows, as well. By filling in her brows slightly, she brought the coloring and contours of her face more into balance.

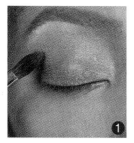

① Using an allover eye shadow brush, apply a light neutral eye shadow all over the lid. This can also be applied to only the upper half of the eyelid.

② Using a crease brush, apply a dark-toned eye shadow (black, brown, blue, purple, or gray) on the lid of the eye only.

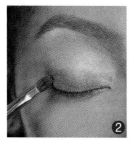

③ Using a blender brush, apply a medium-toned eye shadow to the outer ends of the dark shadow. With back-and-forth strokes, blend and soften the harsh look of the dark shadow. The added eye shadow will also give dimension and the illusion of a crease.

④ Using an eyeliner brush, apply a liquid liner as close to the lash line as possible. (*Tip:* When applying a liquid liner, try beginning the first stroke at the center of the eye's lash line instead of at the inner corner. This is because at times, there might be a thick glob of black liquid on the brush. It is much easier to control, mix, and blend out from the center of the lash line than it would be from a large black smudge at the inner corner of the eye.) Line the bottom of the eye at the lash line with a creamy black pencil.

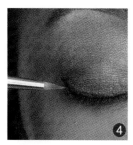

⑤ Using a smudger brush dipped into a dark eye shadow, gently dab over the liquid line just created, which will smoke it out. Try to wait until the liquid liner has dried and set for smoother results. (*Tip:* Smoking out will make eyeliner last longer.)

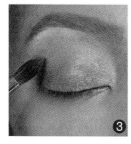

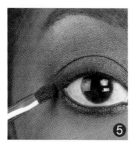

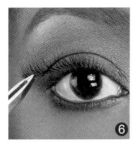

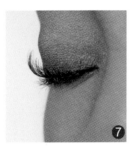

6 Apply false lashes (see the instructions that follow).

7 Let stand and dry (see the instructions that follow).

8 Apply mascara (see the instructions that follow).

9 Using an eyebrow brush, fill in the eyebrows with a light shade (brown, reddish, light brown). Try to avoid using black; it tends to look a bit harsh.

10 Using a smudger brush and a goldish or other shimmery hue, highlight under the dark shadow and along the entire lower lash line and inner eye to soften the makeup and give the eye a bit of sizzle.

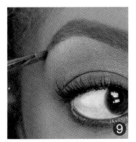

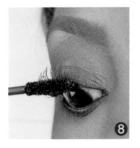

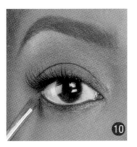

How to Apply False Eyelashes

1. Before applying lashes, remove them from carrying case and with tweezers or fingers remove any of the sticky glue left on the lashes. Next, place the lashes over your own and decide how much of their ends you should cut off. (Brand-new lashes are too long for most people.)
2. Look straight in the mirror, and make sure the lashes begin where the colored part of your eyeball does. This point is about one-fifth of the way from the center edge of the eye to the outer edge.
3. Dab a bit of eyelash glue (I prefer using waterproof) along the inside of a strip's base. Wait fifteen to thirty seconds for the glue to dry slightly.
4. Close your eye slightly and position the false eyelashes over the top of your own lashes. Press the strip of false lashes as close as possible to the roots of your own lashes. Make sure you secure both the inner and outer corners of the false lashes against your own.
5. Keep the eye closed for up to sixty seconds while gently pressing the false eyelashes against the roots of your own. While the lashes are drying, hold them upright against the lid. It will look strange, but trust me: This is the best way to ensure that the eye will appear larger and more open.
6. Apply a coat of mascara on both sides of the lashes. This will blend your own and the false lashes until they become one, achieving a more natural look. To hide the false eyelashes' seam, apply a thin line of liquid eyeliner over their base. (At this point, blending or smoking out again is optional.)

EVE'S TIPS

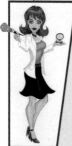

For Eye Shadow and Eyeliner

• When using dark shadows or creating a smoky look, there might be a tendency for the eye shadow to fall on the face, messing up the foundation. You have two options. First, you can apply extra loose powder under your eyes and over your cheekbones to catch the fallout, which you can dust off. Or you can apply the eye makeup first, then clean the excess fallout with a moisturizer and continue with the foundation and rest of the makeup application.

• To apply eyeliner, use a soft pencil liner, pull the lid skin taut, and, getting as close to the lash line as possible, glide the pencil along the upper lid. Try starting at the center, working your way out, and then going back to the inner edge and connecting the line. You can even dab a few dots on the edge of the lash line and then connect them together.

• Apply eye shadow to the crease by looking in the mirror while tipping your head slightly back. Where your eye meets the socket is where the shadow should be lightly swiped.

• To keep your eyes from blinking when applying makeup, try keeping your mouth open—it really works.

Remove Dark Circles Above and Below the Eyes

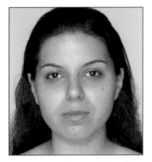

Elena has dark eyes that glisten, but she would like to get rid of dark circles both on top of and beneath her eyes, which not only make her look tired but cause her eyes to look sunken, as well. Opening or extending her eyes will help her achieve a better proportion to her face.

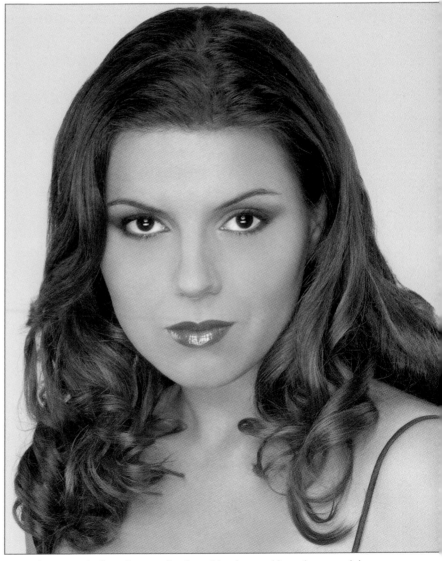

Once Elena smoothed out the overall colors of her face and brought more subtle attention to her beautiful brown eyes, she was able to bring tremendous light and energy into her face.

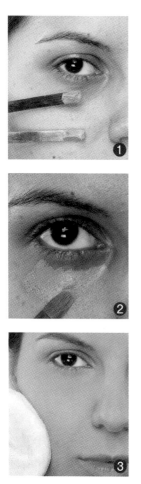

❶ Elena's natural skin tone is olive. To cover up the deep bluish circles, use a light-peach-colored concealer to neutralize the blue. As you can see, it is actually a bit deeper than the olive-colored cream foundation. As with all of us, the skin underneath Elena's eyes is thinner than the rest of her face, and sometimes can reveal a slightly bluish color, which is made up of a combination of veins, blood, and pigment showing through the skin. Using the salmon color, even if it appears darker than the foundation, will even out the blue and will easily blend into the foundation.

❷ Using a concealer brush, apply the concealer underneath the eye and on the eyelid. Avoid applying too much concealer in the eye area or placing it too close to the rim of the eye. Instead, use the excess left on the sponge when blending it in to cover the delicate areas underneath and above the lid. A little concealer goes a long way. This will prevent caking up and creasing of excess product.

❸ With a sponge, apply the foundation. (Either liquid or cream foundation will work.) Blend the foundation with the concealer by gently patting the foundation over the concealer and smoothing the line between the two. Applying loose translucent powder with either a powder puff or a powder brush, set the foundation.
    Proceed with regular makeup application.

For a Quick Touch-Up

If, after a long day, you find that the makeup under your eyes has caked or smudged, use a makeup sponge with some moisturizer or a baby-wipe-type makeup remover in the area under the eyes. Let it dry, then reapply the concealer, foundation, or powder, and blend into the rest of the face.

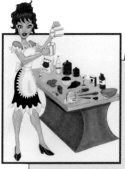

- **Wet, used tea bags (inexpensive nonherbal):** These act as a poultice, drawing out excess fluids while refreshing and soothing the eye area. The tea contains tannic acid, an antioxidant.
- **Raw potato slices:** They will take away dark circles under the eyes (potatoes contain potassium).
- **Cucumber slices:** These draw out excess fluids, reducing baggy eyes.
- **Anbesol:** When tweezing eyebrows, Anbesol will numb the brow area and spare you from the pain.
- **Toothbrush and hair spray:** Use to tame those unruly brows.
- **Eyedrops:** Use to remove redness not only from your eyes but also from red blemishes.
- **Preparation H:** This will relieve puffiness around the eyes and tighten skin. You can mix Preparation H with moisturizer to mask the medicinal odor.

Tools for Your Eyes

- Concealer, foundation, sponge
- Loose powder, powder puff
- Brushes: concealer, allover eyelid, eye blender, eye definer, eye smudger, eyeliner, eyebrow, spooly
- Lash separator
- Eyelash curler, mascara, fake lashes, glue
- Eyeliners
- Eye shadows

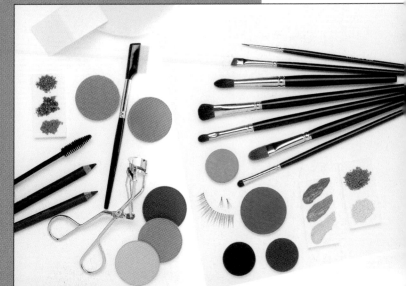

The key to flawless-looking makeup is blending. Eliminating hard lines around the eyes, lips, or cheeks is extremely important—it's the art of makeup. These tools (and others mentioned in chapter 7) will help you achieve the look you want.

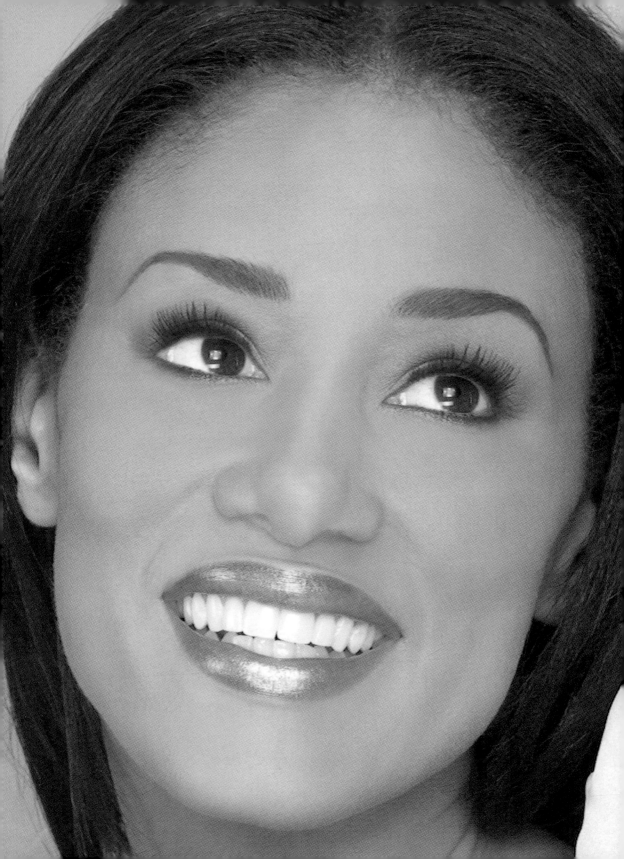

artfully reshape your nose

MAKING THE MOST OF YOUR MOST PROMINENT FEATURE

Aside from its blatant existence, few things are plain about the nose.
It is esthetically deceptive, symbolically bipolar, physically protean,
and even semi-secessionist.

Daniel McNeill, *The Face*

The nose is the seat of the face's power. No matter who you are, it sits in the center of your face and is your most prominent feature. This is true whether you have a pug nose, one that turns up at the end, one that is long and angular, one that has a slight bump on the ridge, or one with larger-than-average nostrils. And even those of us born with a small, button nose are often unhappy with its shape, size, or look. The evidence of this discomfort lies in the fact that one of the five most popular plastic surgery procedures is rhinoplasty—in short, the nose job.

Because rhinoplasty is so common among both women and men, many people think that there is no risk involved. But think again. Chances are, you will experience one or more of the risks of surgery: bleeding, swelling, and, in some cases, a new nose that you are not happy with. And then there's the cost, which averages $3,500—and often even more.

So why take any risks at all when you can accomplish the same goals with makeup? Using makeup, you can attain your idealized nose, steer clear of both the risks and costs of surgery, and avoid the possible disappointment or regret of a permanent change.

If you really look at your face, you'll see the uniqueness and beauty of your not-perfectly-straight or bold Roman nose. Then you'll begin to see how in fact the shape of your nose actually fits you *perfectly,* as it is aligned to accentuate all of your fabulous facial features. Your maker knew what she was doing when she created you!

So just as you have with your other features, have fun with your nose—celebrate it. Let it be big and bold one day, small and delicate the next, and fiery aquiline another. Using makeup, you can do whatever you choose—just take a look at Iteka and Claudia below.

The Dangers of Rhinoplasty

While rhinoplasty—plastic surgery of the nose—has vastly improved over the past twenty-five years, there are always some potential dangers the patient may face, including bleeding, infection, or anesthetic problems that, in the worst-case scenario, can result in death. People have also reported losing their sense of smell. And then there is another downside: the cost. The average rhinoplasty costs $3,500.

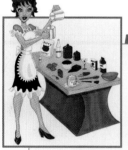

EVE'S HOME REMEDIES

- **Eyedrops** will remove redness not only from your eyes but also from red blemishes. Freeze a drop in a spoon, place it frozen over the blemish, and hold. It will shrink swelling.
- **Neosporin** can help heal and remove acne overnight.
- **Toothpaste** (white paste) will help heal acne breakouts.
- **Clay masks** will draw out the blackheads that tend to gather around the nose. They work by dehydrating the top layer of skin.
- **Cuticle scissors** work well to trim those little nose hairs.

Straightening the Nose

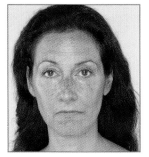

You may remember Claudia from the eye chapter, where we hid her crow's-feet and highlighted the natural glow of her skin by evening out her skin tone. In the shots that follow, you can see how we deemphasized a bump on Claudia's otherwise beautiful nose.

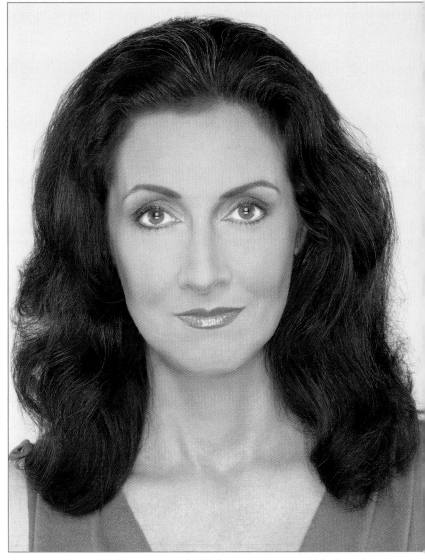

Claudia is an example of how makeup highlights certain features while deemphasizing others, creating a dramatic whole. Rather than covering the natural luminescence of her skin, the makeup actually lets it shine through.

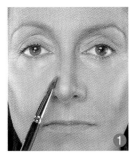

1. Using a thin, flat concealer brush with a cream foundation two tones darker than the skin color, shade the sides of the nose to even out the bump. When contouring a nose that's broken, is crooked, or has a bump, look straight in the mirror. Begin the shading at the inner edge of the lashes and, while working down toward the nostrils, adjust the shading area to create the illusion of a straight nose. Then, with a clean brush or a sponge, blend out and soften any harsh contour lines.

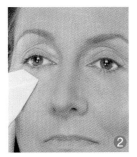

2. Using a makeup sponge or a powder puff, apply loose powder to set the foundation. When powdering around areas with contouring, pat gently with the loose powder. (*Tip:* When using a powder puff, try to apply the powder in one circular motion by placing the puff down on one side and rotating it to the other. Then lift the puff straight off. This will prevent rubbing off the contouring.)

The contour shading can be applied using a brown or taupe eye or blush shadow and an edged contour brush. Place the brush in the shadow, dust off any excess, and apply the brush using thin strokes along the sides of the nose. Be cautious with dry powder around the nose, so it doesn't look dirty.

A Thinner, Smaller Nose

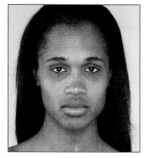

Though Iteka likes most of her features, she has always felt that her nose is too wide. I think her nose not only fits her face, but also reveals an inner strength of character. If, like Iteka, you sometimes prefer to make your nose look thinner or smaller, follow these five easy steps. Note that as we thinned the shape of her nose, we also deemphasized some of the blotchiness of her skin.

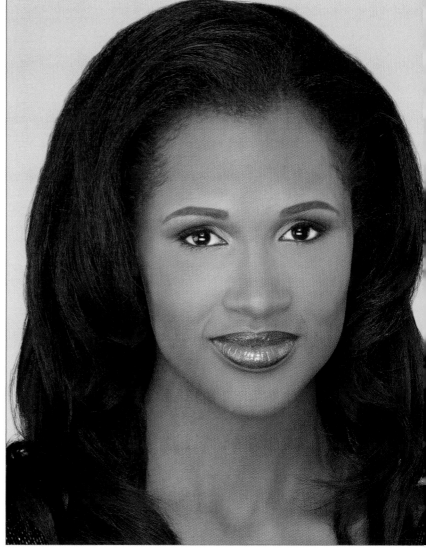

These simple steps help Iteka achieve the look she wants—a slightly thinner nose. As you can see, Iteka clearly possesses an exotic beauty, enhanced by the quick makeup tips that follow.

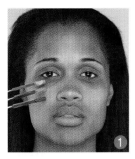

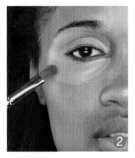

1 Here we used three shades of concealing cream foundation— a light-honey-toned shade to cover the undereye circles and the T-zone, a medium shade to use all around the face, and a dark shade to contour and thin out the nose. Regardless of the color or tone of your skin, the general guidelines for creating contour remain the same for the nose: You use three colors to create the shading effect. One color matches your skin tone; one color is a shade or two lighter to highlight particular areas; and one color is a shade or two darker to define certain areas, as when thinning out a nose or even distracting the eye from a slightly crooked nose.

2 Using a concealer brush, apply the yellow-honey (the shade closest to your skin color) concealing foundation on the dark areas around the eyes.

3 With a sponge, apply the medium shade of foundation and blend it together with the lighter shade using a gentle patting motion where the two shades meet.

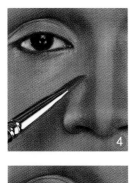

④ With a thin, flat concealer brush, apply the dark shade around the side edges of the nose. Begin at the inner corners of the eyebrows and brush straight down to the nostrils.

⑤ At first the lines drawn on the edges appear quite harsh, and since railroad tracks are not attractive on your nose, it's best to blend them out. With a sponge or a clean brush, blend out the edges to soften the lines. Apply powder to set.

As you can see with Iteka and Claudia in this chapter, you have the power and the tools to fashion the nose you wish. Using just a concealer, foundation, and contour brush, you can work small miracles! Now you are ready to use makeup to highlight or deemphasize your nose. And then when you're bored, you can remove the makeup and try something else out for size!

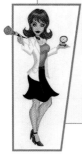

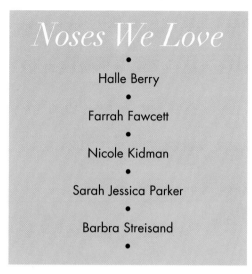

Noses We Love

- Halle Berry
- Farrah Fawcett
- Nicole Kidman
- Sarah Jessica Parker
- Barbra Streisand

Tools for Your Nose

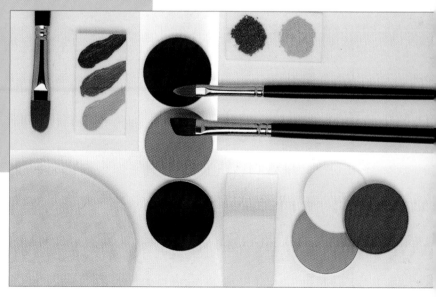

- Sponge
- Powder puff
- Brushes: concealer, small-edged contour
- Concealers
- Foundation
- Loose powders
- Contouring shadows

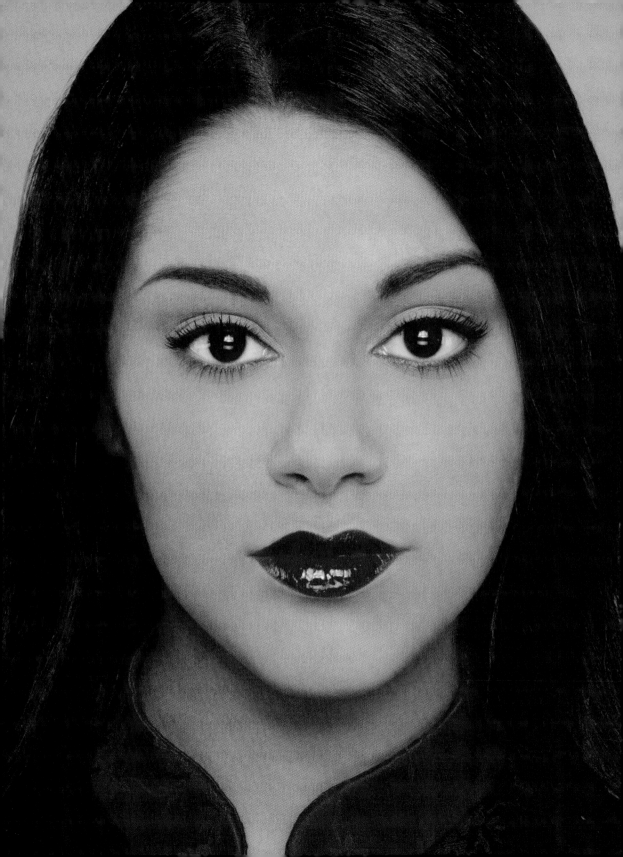

your
lips
THE SPICE OF THE FACE

Lips are the spice of the face,
twin ruddy bulges separated by the dark line of the mouth,
like a pair of cushions.
Daniel McNeill, *The Face*

There is probably no feature more significant and important for a woman then her lips. Luscious, pouty, and sexy, a woman's lips are the gateway to her two most seductive sources of power: her sensuality and her voice.

For centuries, women have wielded power through the kiss. Her decision whether or not to allow a man to kiss her was often a woman's only source of leverage, of power, in a world ruled by men. And like women, lips are complex. One day, they're forceful, forming words that reverberate and transform lives. The next, they are soft and supple, inviting and promising. They want to get dressed up and look pretty. *They want to seduce.* Did you know that lips become flushed and rosy when we're sexually aroused? That's why we wear lip color—to mimic this effect.

Indeed, the art of seduction begins with a woman's lips, so it is not surprising that throughout the ages women have been very preoccupied with how to best present their smackers. Who can forget the Roaring Twenties when adorning lips with vibrant shades of red became all the rage? This was also the era when the "bow" lips of screen siren Clara Bow became famous. Childlike yet womanly, Clara Bow radiated sex appeal. Following her trend, another pair of sexy lips emerged on the scene, this time on cartoon goddess Betty Boop. Her surname was even added to emphasize her lips: Each time she rendered her signature line, "Boop-boop-bee-doop," she brought attention to her mouth and lips, asking her audience to kiss her.

In the 1940s, lips were played down. In the 1950s, pale, shimmering, ultrafeminine lipsticks were introduced into the marketplace; by the 1960s, shades of pink had become the rage. The women's movement in the 1970s heralded a more natural look, and while some fashionistas espoused this earthy look well into the 1980s, many women were also donning power suits. They made a stronger statement with their mouths as well as their brains—fire-engine red became the unofficial power color of this decade.

By the 1990s, power suits were out, but big, pouty, sultry lips and myriad colors to decorate them were—and still are—in. Think of Michelle Pfeiffer, Angelina Jolie, Madonna, or Julia Roberts—to name just a few. With this rage for large, pouty lips has come a dramatic increase in surgery and other treatments to attain the desired effect. Now when we flip through the glossy mags, we are often drawn in by the question and the mystery behind the Hollywood stars' lips: Are they God-given or doctor-enhanced?

In the past decade, thousands of women each year decide to plump their lips, investing in a procedure known as lip augmentation, with 60 percent of the patients being younger than fifty. Although considered generally safe, lip enlargement, as with any surgical procedure, involves certain risks, such as ulceration or scarring. In a rare and very extreme case, a woman with collagen lip injections was traveling on an airplane when a drop in air pressure caused her lips to explode! More realistic risks include a literally stiff upper lip—swelling (who can forget Goldie Hawn's character's lips in the film *The First Wives Club*!) or hard lips that feel unnatural to touch or kiss. Also possible are allergic reactions, drooling, unnatural movement when talking or smiling, infection, and poorly placed lips.

The most popular substance used to inject lips is collagen—which, to put it bluntly, is just another term for "cow skin." Another is called Dermalogen, aka human cadaver skin. Other substances that can be used include the fat from an area of the patient's own body, usually the groin, and Gore-Tex, a synthetic material that is normally used to keep us dry when it's raining!

Some women feel a certain reluctance or downright refusal to partake in the quest for perfect lips once they discover what those larger-than-life sexy smackers are really made of, not to mention how painful the procedure is and how often it needs to be done to maintain the look—usually every four to six months. Instead of going to such lengths, why not try a simpler approach? The next time you feel the urge to enlarge, make more shapely, or even minimize your lips, use these makeup techniques instead.

Check out the three women you'll see in this chapter. As you'll learn, not only is it possible to attain your ideal lips using a few tried-and-true techniques, but you can also choose the color you feel best suits them—*your own* ideal color. And what's ideal for you? Whatever color makes you feel most beautiful when you walk out the front door.

The Risks and the Costs of Lip Augmentation

Many women opt for cosmetic surgery to augment their lips, but before you make a decision, consider these facts. For starters, the cost can be astronomical. Depending on the amount of collagen injected, the price can range from $400 to $7,000—and the procedure usually lasts only four to six months. And remember, these estimates do not include medical tests, prescriptions, or facility and anesthesiologist costs. There are also costs besides the monetary one: While the risk is low, women may still experience infection, numbing, scarring, swelling, stiffness in the lips, distorted lips, and an adverse, potentially deadly reaction to anesthesia.

Luscious—but Smaller—Lips

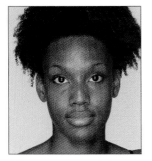

Tiffany was born with large lips that have a luscious quality—something a lot of women would kill for, or at least pay a lot of money! Certainly many Hollywood stars have. But just as so many of us become bored with whatever Mother Nature has endowed us with, Tiffany is tired of her bodacious lips and wants to tone down their size. For her, less is best. Here are a few simple tips that will help make her (and your!) lips appear smaller.

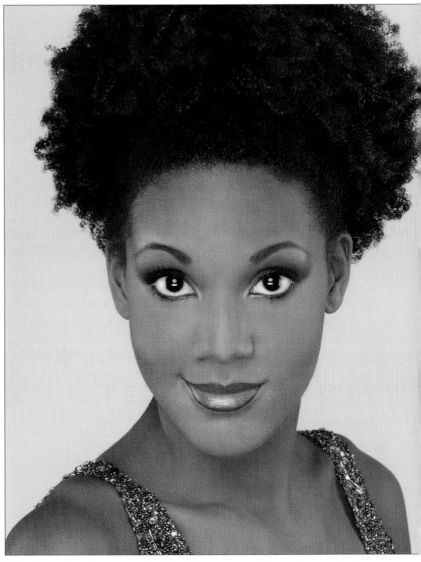

Tiffany's transformation is complete! Her lips appear smaller, and seem to balance the dramatic arch of her brows with the rest of her features.

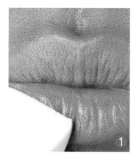

1 Using a sponge, apply foundation all over the lips. This will create a sort of blank canvas. (Think of Japanese Kabuki makeup, which whites out the entire face and then re-creates the features.)

2 Powder the entirety of your lips to help set the foundation for the lipstick. This way, what you put on, stays on.

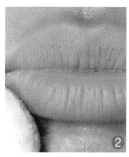

3 Using a lip pencil, outline the size (and shape) of the lips that you would like to have. This may feel a little strange at first if you're used to outlining the full circumference of your lips, but don't worry—you'll be thrilled when you see the final result. For best results, from the top and bottom, outline the inside one-quarter of your lips—or even less, as done here with Tiffany. (*Tip:* You can eliminate this step if you use a nude lip gloss.) The purpose of outlining the lips in this way is to give them definition. Try to use a neutral tone for outlining, such as a shade of taupe, mahogany, or wine.

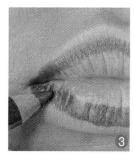

4 Using a lip brush, apply either a lipstick or a gloss around the inside lip area. With the lip brush, go over the lip liner to blend out any hard edge left behind from the pencil. I prefer using warm, light shades in peach, nude, gold. But any shade you are comfortable with will work.

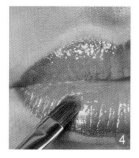

Here's how to prevent lipstick from getting on your teeth. After applying lipstick and/or gloss, place your finger into your mouth, wrap your lips around the finger, and gently pull it out in a lollipop motion. The excess lipstick on the inside of your lips will end up on your finger instead of your teeth. Simply wipe it off on a tissue and you're set to go.

A Plumper Upper Lip

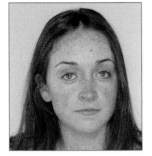

Colleen has small, delicate lips. She longs for a fuller top lip, as well as a "sweetheart" shape to her lips. The first step toward achieving this effect is to apply foundation and powder—the same products you used for the rest of your face—on top of and around the lip area. This process acts like a primer, holding and maintaining the lip color much longer. It will also eliminate losing the inner color and being left with that distracting line around your mouth that's so dismaying when you look at yourself in the bathroom mirror after you've just finished that drink with your date!

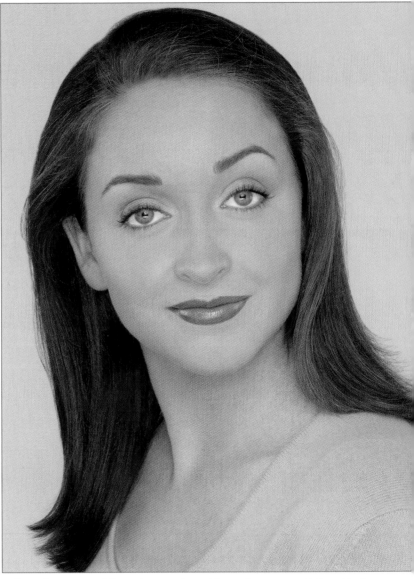

Colleen's lips are now fuller and more sultry, adding to her more sophisticated look.

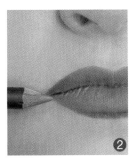

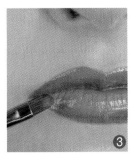

1 Using a lip pencil, outline the desired shape and size of the top and bottom lips. It's easy to create a heart shape, as on Colleen, just by using the pencil to round out (or slightly expand) the top edges and the bottom lip. At the same time, you are also naturally increasing the appearance of your lips, making them seem more pronounced.

2 Now fill in the entire area with the pencil. This will create another layer that also helps keep the color on the lips longer and maintains a look that's natural for the lip size.

3 For the final step, fill in the lips with a lip gloss to create a moist, plump look. Note that a light-tinted gloss will add another dimension, making the lips "pop"!

Reshaping the Lips
(and Preventing Color from Bleeding)

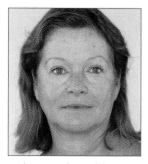

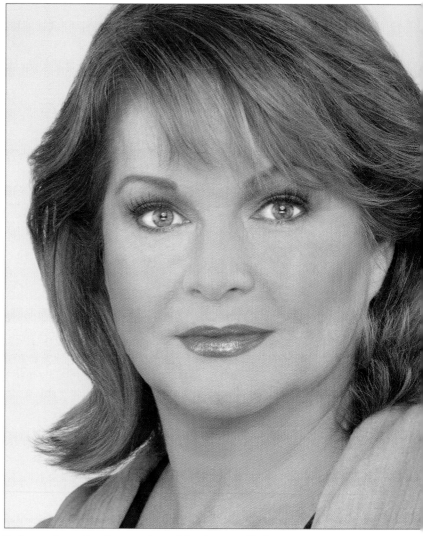

Barbara is a beautiful woman whose natural bone structure gives her built-in strength to fight the effects of aging. But like so many women, she wished to adjust the slight unevenness of her lips. She also wanted to feel confident that her lipstick would stay on her lips and not feather or bleed into any fine lines around her mouth. It didn't take long for her to become convinced of makeup's power to make her look and feel much more confident and younger! Watch how a few simple makeup techniques create a fabulous end result.

Barbara enlarged her lips, creating a fuller shape and balancing out any unevenness. Also, she was able to eliminate any feathering around the lips, which used to cause her lipstick to bleed. Do I need to mention that Barbara has been converted—to makeup, that is! The beauty that defines her now shines—from both inside and out. She looks radiant and youthful, and those lips are perky!

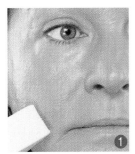

① Using a sponge, apply a sheer cream foundation to the face as well as over the lips.

② Using a powder puff, apply loose powder to set the foundation over the face and the lips. This process will create a primer over the lips and hold the lipstick better.

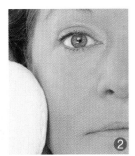

③ Using a pencil with a shade similar to whatever lip color will top it—or at least in the same family—create the desired size and shape for the lips. Try to round off the top edges and curve the bottom lip. When increasing the size of the lips, avoid making them too wide. Instead, increase the size with a move that rounds off rather than widens out, which is more complimentary and youthful looking.

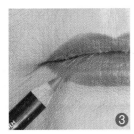

④ If you make a mistake, don't panic. Simply take a concealer brush and, using either concealer or foundation and a small, light back-and-forth motion, correct the area with excess lip liner. Working it all around the edges will actually smooth out that line and fill in any feathering lines around the lip area. (This process works just like an eraser.)

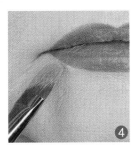

⑤ Using a wedge makeup sponge, apply loose powder around the edges of the lips. Don't be stingy; apply the powder all around in order to set the lips and fill in the ridges, which will prevent the lipstick from bleeding downward. Then wipe off any excess with either the back of the wedge or a brush.

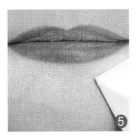

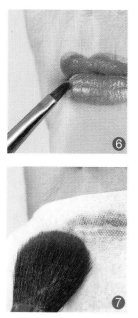

⑥ Apply a lipstick similar in color to the lip liner.

⑦ To set that lipstick and keep it in place, separate a tissue, place one sheet on top of the lips, and dab on loose powder with a powder brush. Then repeat the lipstick. This will help keep that lipstick in place, even after you've had a few nibbles or a drink! To add dimension, applying a light shimmery gloss over the lipstick will make lips "pop."

For everyday wear, choose lip color in neutral shades such as mauve (a pink-and-orange combination). Also, when choosing a lip texture, keep in mind that a matte lipstick has more pigment (color) and stays on longer than the sheer or glossy kind. You can always apply a gloss over the lipstick for added shine.

EVE'S TIPS

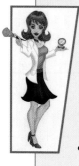

Hot Lip Tips

- The same way you clean out your closets, clean out your makeup bag. Get rid of that lipstick you spent a fortune on but makes you look like a clown or a vampire.
- Next time, buy yourself that sexy lipstick.
- Apply lip liner all over the lip and then top off with a gloss . . . it lasts longer.
- For a natural look, outline your lips with a color that is *lighter* than your lipstick.

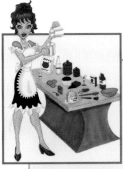

- **Jell-O:** Dab a Q-tip into cherry-flavored Jell-O powder and apply to your lips. Let it sit for five minutes, then lick it off. This will give your lips a natural red coat.
- **Toothbrush and Vaseline:** Use these to exfoliate and plump up your lips.
- **Eucerin lotion:** Apply over your lips for soothing therapy and to hold lip color.
- **Yellow eye shadow:** Try applying a yellow eye shadow as a primer on your lips. It will warm up any lip color.
- **Vaseline** added to any shadow can make a gel blush or lip stain.
- **Parsley** will help freshen your breath from the inside. Parsley contains chlorophyll, which is also found in Certs and Clorets.

Tools for Your Lips

- Sponge
- Concealer
- Foundation
- Powder puff
- Powder
- Brushes: concealer, lip, powder
- Lip liners
- Lipstick
- Lip gloss
- Tissue

As the adage goes, sometimes, pictures speak louder than words—just look at the before and after shots of Colleen, Tiffany, and Barbara. Using only a few simple tools, including the wedge, lip pencil, foundation, and concealer, these three women's mouths—and therefore their faces—were transformed. And you can do the same today. Enjoy!

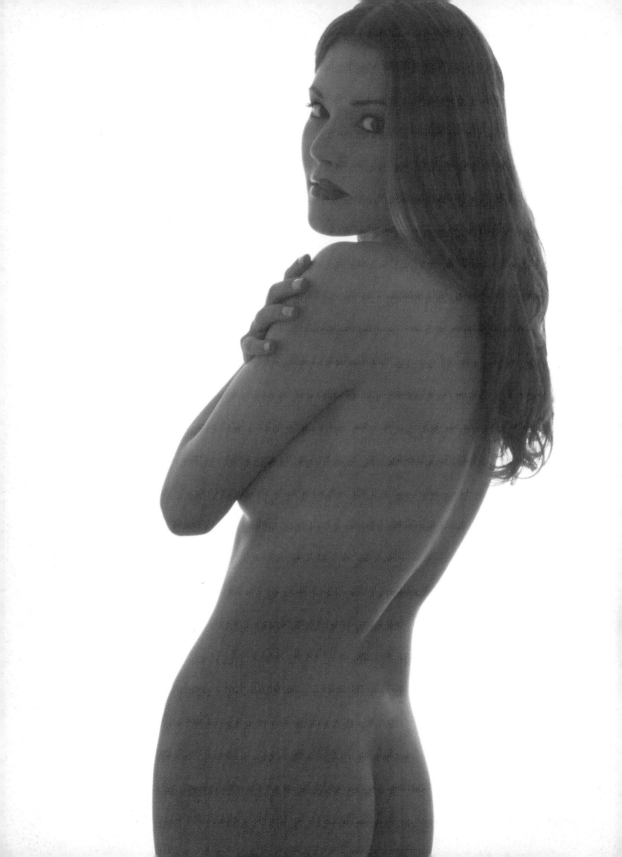

breast

& body

THE QUEST FOR PERFECTION

I sing the body electric

Walt Whitman

The Breasts

The quest for the "perfect" breasts has become a near obsession in our country over the past few decades—just flip through any magazine or watch any soap opera. These women seem to be flaunting perfectly shaped, sized, and perched breasts for all the world to see. But in many cases, what we are seeing isn't natural. These breasts have a sculpted look because they *have been* sculpted—injected with silicone and saline, or propped up with muscle tissue from other areas of the body (most notably the derrière), and manipulated to hang a certain number of perfect inches above the belly button and below eye level.

Another sign that America is looking outward to feel better inward, and many women are willing to go under the knife to get what they want.

Today's media seem obsessed with women and their breasts. We are deluged with images of the voluptuous profiles of stars such as Pamela Anderson, Salma Hayek, and Halle Berry, causing many an American woman to feel she needs bigger, better breasts. Combine this pressure with technological advances in plastic surgery and you've got the beginning of a craze. There is also the regret syndrome: Many women who get plastic surgery mourn for their original breasts, as though they have left behind a crucial part of what makes them unique.

Besides not feeding your soul, plastic surgery for the breasts is not completely safe. There are still many outstanding questions. First, experts wonder about potential adverse long-term effects of implants. Second, doctors warn that with implants, cancerous lumps may be more difficult to detect on routine mammograms. Breast implants may also negatively impact a woman's ability to breast-feed. And finally, while many people think that implantation is a one-shot deal, the procedure must often be repeated when the material used for augmentation begins to disintegrate internally or move. Furthermore, the saline solution used for implantation has been known to burst or wear over time—not to mention that you may experience an increase or decrease in breast sensation after surgery. And, as with any surgical procedure, there are the "standard" risks from anesthesia, infection, swelling, redness, bleeding, and pain. Implants can also leak, harden, leave scars, and cause you to lose sensitivity. The potential risks of breast reduction are also significant: Many women complain that they have lost all sensation in their breasts. Although reduction surgery is often covered by insurance, it can range from $4,000 to $10,000.

Why risk these potential dangers and costs when you can enlarge your breasts with makeup and a few of our other handy-dandy tricks? With makeup, you risk nothing because it's temporary! For the record, Julia Roberts gives credit to her enhanced breasts for helping her win an Academy Award for *Erin Brockovich*. And Julia did it all without surgery!

Potential Dangers of Breast Surgery

- Implants can obscure the results of mammography.

- Any reduction or enlargement of the breast can prevent nursing an infant.

- Undergoing any surgical procedure involves the risk of complications such as anesthesia reactions, infection, swelling, redness, bleeding, and pain.

- There is also a risk of deflation or rupture of the saline-solution-filled breast implants. This requires additional surgery to remove and possibly replace the implants.

- According to the Food and Drug Administration, there is "a high chance that you will need to have additional surgery at some point to replace or remove the implant. Also, problems such as deflation, capsular contracture, infection, shifting, and calcium deposits can require removal of the implants."

- Once breasts are enlarged with injections, self-examination becomes more difficult.

- You may experience physical pain for days or even months following the procedure.

- You may experience an increase or loss of sensitivity in your breasts—and keep in mind that they're an erogenous zone.

- For more information on the dangers of breast augmentation, visit the FDA's Web site (www.fda.gov).

Breast Enlargement

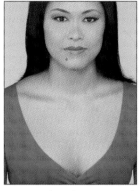

Sung Yun has always wanted to increase her breast size. Here, I am going to show the best way to change from an A cup to a B or C cup. All you need are a few strokes of a brush and the magic of the Wonderbra (or any similar padded and uplifting bra).

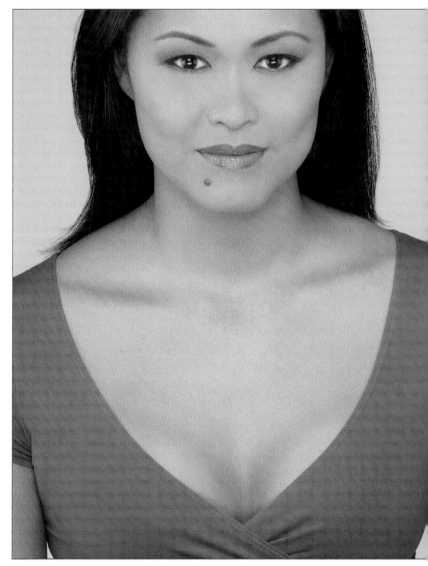

I must say, I've never seen Sung Yun more excited than when she began to see her breasts transform from pretty and pert to absolutely voluptuous! It's a simple trick of the trade that is easy to do and looks completely natural.

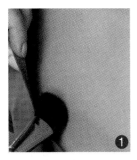

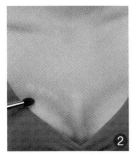

❶ In this photo, Sung Yun is wearing her Wonderbra. Begin by using an eye or blush shadow two shades darker than your own skin tone. In this case, I used taupe, the same color I used to contour Sung Yun's cheeks. A bronzer can also be used for this process, as long as it is not too shiny. Using an angled blush brush, make back-and-forth strokes (think of windshield-wiper strokes) beginning at the inner part between the breasts and ending at the top of the breast, near the clothing area. (*Tip:* Make sure to lightly apply the dark contour shadow.)

❷ Highlight with a shadow color (eye shadow or blush) that's two shades lighter than your own skin color (try ivory, white, vanilla). With a long contour brush, apply the highlighter between the breasts, as well as both above and below the dark shadow. This motion is to blend out the darker shadow and create dimensions in the rounding of the breasts.

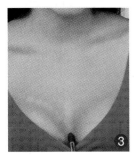

❸ Continue the shading and highlighting process once or twice more to achieve as natural or intense a look as you desire.

Emphasize Cleavage

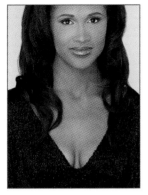

Iteka is comfortable with her B-size breasts, but on special nights, she'd like to add a little oomph. Take a look at how we perked them up a bit.

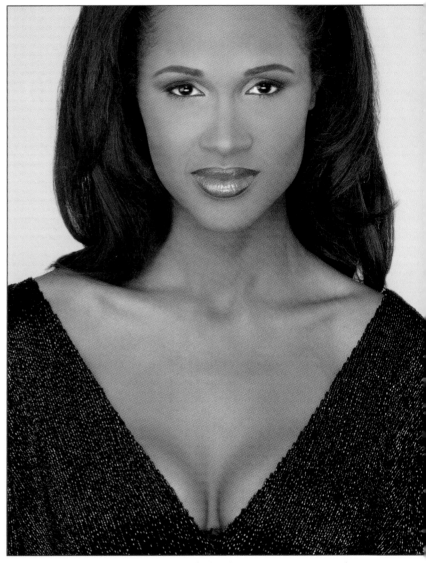

I would say Iteka looks swell in this beautiful black dress. As you can see, this process actually makes her breasts appear an entire bra size larger—with only a few quick strokes!

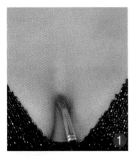

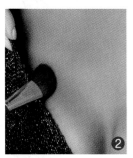

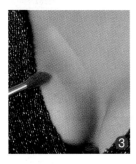

1 The first step is to put on a Wonderbra or similar padded, uplift-style bra. We then used a highlight color one or two shades lighter than Iteka's skin tone. (You can use either eye shadow or blush colors of yellow, ivory, or off-white.) With a vertical up-and-down motion and a long blender brush, apply the shade between the breasts.

2 Next, use an angled shadow brush and a blusher or eye shadow that's two tones darker than your own (taupe, brown, or bronze—just adjust intensity depending on your skin tone). With rounded back-and-forth motions (again, almost like a windshield wiper), begin lightly applying the shadow to the upper breast area. Begin and end the stroke inside the clothing area. (*Tip:* It is better to go farther in than risk the possibility of your top moving and having a shadow edge showing.)

3 Using the long blender brush, apply the highlighter above and below the dark shadow area and again in the center.

Continue this process until you achieve a smooth, effective look. Be sure to blend. In this case, less is more. A little shadow and highlight go a long way. You can also use some bronzer powder all over and a highlight shimmer powder between the breasts.

A Breast and Bra Time Line

- 2500 B.C. In Crete, Greece, the first corset (made out of some sort of fabric, it is believed) is invented.

- A.D. 1550. A woman named Catherine de Médicis, wife of King Henry II of France during the 1550s, supposedly invents the first steel corset.

- Circa 1650. Apparently, Louis XIV of France insists on "lower necklines" for all the women in his court, setting the fashion across the Western world.

- 1893. Marie Tucek creates the first modern brassiere, called the "breast supporter."

- 1914. Mary Phelps Jacobs is credited for patenting the brassiere. (Marie Tucek's choice, *breast supporter*, is changed apparently because it is not politically correct.)

- 1917. The brassiere officially replaces the corset. The U.S. War Industries Board calls on women to cease buying corsets apparently because it needs the metal for the war effort.

- 1920s, the flapper era. Legs are in, as well as smaller breasts.

- 1930s, the Great Depression. Backs are in. Smaller breasts remain popular, although larger breasts are slowly starting to come back into fashion.

- 1940s, World War II. Security, apple pie, and big-breasted women are in.

- 1950s. Big breasts are still in.

- 1960s and 1970s. The women's movement, the sexual revolution, and civil rights herald a more natural look. If anything, flatter is better.

- 1980s and on up to today. Reagan, conservatism, and objectification of the breast come back into style. Technological advances in plastic surgery make it possible for many American women to get breast augmentation.

Tools for Your Breasts

- Brushes: blush, angled blush, long blender blush
- Shadows (can be blush or eye shadows): taupe, deep brown, off-white, yellow, bronzer
- A Wonderbra or similar padded, uplifting bra

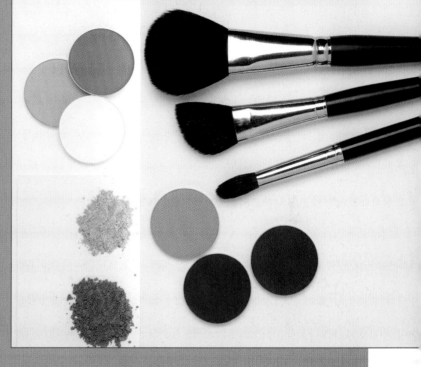

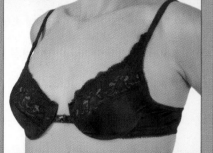

Other bra

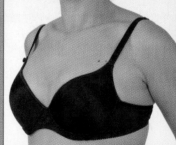

Wonderbra

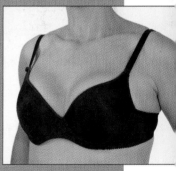

Wonderbra and shading

The Body

Like even the most beloved car, our bodies can take a beating from the general wear and tear of driving through life. Growing up, we first encounter pimples, sometimes acne, and it is difficult to get through our teens without a few scars from playing field hockey or getting a tattoo. As we get older, the skin of our body naturally begins to lose its elasticity, tone, and firmness, so that by the time we're in our thirties and forties, age spots, red blotches, and other marks appear as if out of nowhere.

Whether caused by our lifestyle, genetics, or the inevitable passage of time, signs of aging and marks caused by the sun—or a wild trip to the tattoo parlor—begin to bother us. Many women and men eventually decide they don't want to look at them any longer. But what are their options? Of course, some people decide to remove their scars, age spots, or tattoos through such popular procedures as laser surgery, dermabrasion, and chemical peels. But all have their risks; laser surgery, for instance, can actually burn the skin.

There is also risk related to the person who actually performs the surgery. The Food and Drug Administration regulates which lasers are on the market but does not regulate how the physician carries out the surgery, and people performing these procedures are often not adequately trained. People with sensitive skin are also at special risk. For these people, laser surgery is not a safe bet because their skin may not be able to handle the topical cream they need to apply after the surgery is completed. In other words, you could end up looking a whole lot worse than before you had the surgery.

The Downside of Laser Surgery and Other Procedures

- Laser surgery involves the risk of burning the skin.
- Pigmentation or discoloration can occur—either lighter or darker. For darker-skinned people, it is common for the surgery to cause their skin to become lighter.
- Additional follow-up surgery is often needed.
- For people with sensitive skin, the topical après-surgery creams may cause a reaction or outbreak.
- It takes about ten days to heal after surgery, with the face often covered with blisters, redness, or the like.
- Makeup cannot be worn during the ten-day healing process after surgery.
- It's costly. Although the costs vary, reflecting how big an area needs lasering and how many times the procedure must be repeated, procedures begin at $200 (for removal of a blood vessel from the face) and end near $2,000 (for a large tattoo).
- Collagen can cause an allergic reaction.
- Lasering of dark spots can create a burnlike effect and take weeks to heal.
- You cannot be exposed to sunlight for weeks after many procedures.

Cover Up Tattoos, Bruises, or Hickeys

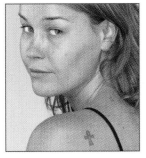

Deirdre is quite fond of the small cross tattoo that sits demurely on the back of her left shoulder. At times, however, she wants the option of not having it there. Instead of permanent removal with laser surgery, makeup will provide more options. You can use the same process to cover up bruises—or even hickeys.

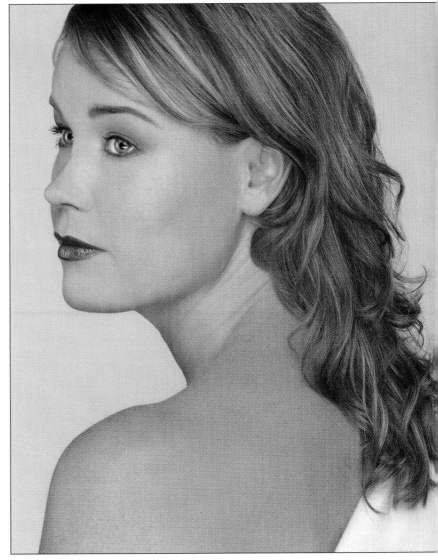

As you can see from the after photo, Deirdre's tattoo is nowhere in sight. Now all that remains are her fair complexion and all-American good looks, simply enhanced with makeup.

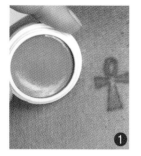

1 Begin by using a salmon or light peach concealer to neutralize the blue of the tattoo; this is the same shade you can use to cover up bluish undereye circles.

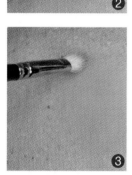

2 Using a concealer brush, apply the light peach shade to the desired area.

3 Use a sponge or a concealer brush to blend the edges into the surrounding skin. This is to avoid having one area look very different from the rest of the skin.

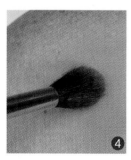

4 Using a powder brush or powder puff, apply loose powder in a patting motion over the covered area to set. There might be a lingering bit of tattoo still showing after you powder, which is okay—you have now created your first layer.

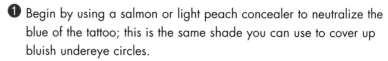

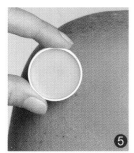

5 The tattoo has now been covered, leaving a patch on Deirdre's shoulder. A lighter color needs to be added to make the area look like real skin. Since Deirdre's natural skin tone is light ivory, a similar light concealer is used.

6 Using a mixing or concealer brush, apply the lighter concealer shade sporadically to areas around the edges and in the center of the area being covered.

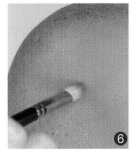

7 Notice the difference in the two shades being used. The two concealer colors will help the area being covered look more like real skin.

8 Using a powder puff or powder brush, apply loose powder to the entire area to set the makeup. Depending on the size or intensity of the tattoo (colors, space, and so forth), repeat these steps as much as needed to cover the area. Remember, as long as you mix several concealer shades together, the outcome will look like real skin. Repeating the powdering will also help set the makeup and keep it there. Dab with a tissue to remove excess oils or powder.

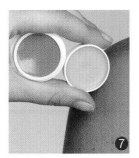

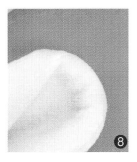

Cover Up II

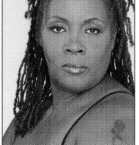

Shirley is unquestionably proud of her rose tattoo. Like Deirdre, however, she likes to hide it at times—especially on nights when she gets dressed up for that black-tie dinner or has a meeting with her boss.

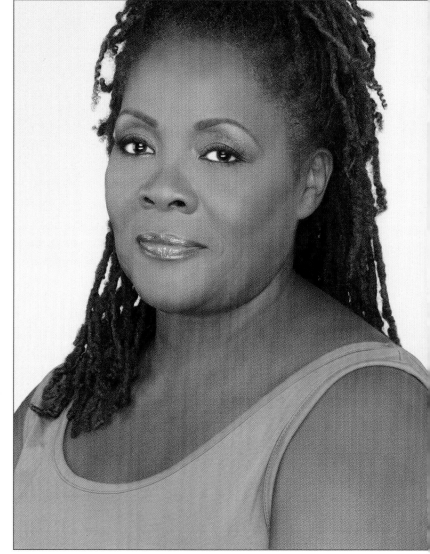

As you can see, Shirley has temporarily removed her tattoo using the same process as Deirdre.

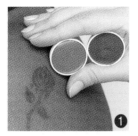

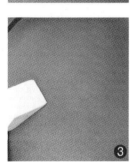

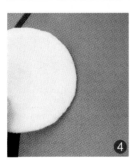

❶ Remember, this process is all about making the tattoo disappear. When covering tattoos (or a bruise or hickey), use two shades of concealer to make the area look more real—like the rest of the skin—instead of one patch of color.

❷ Here, I'm using a light shade in a yellow-honey tone and a medium brown shade to match Shirley's skin tone.

❸ You can also apply the light and dark at once before applying your first coat of loose powder. Try not to rub the concealers off or mix them together. Sporadic light and dark will look much more like real skin than will a blotch of color.

❹ Repeat the process as necessary. This will actually set the makeup in place and create a barrier so that it won't rub off. The key to remember is combining the two shades to make it look like real skin. Dab with a tissue to remove excess oils or powder.

Good-Bye Age and Sun Spots

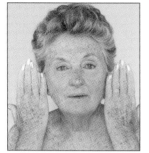

Mary, like many women her age, has age and sun spots on her face, hands, and other parts of the body that are often on display. We want to help cover up these marks while accentuating Mary's natural, lovely features. Instead of laser surgery on the sun and age spots and collagen or fat injections in her hands, however, a few dabs of makeup will do the trick.

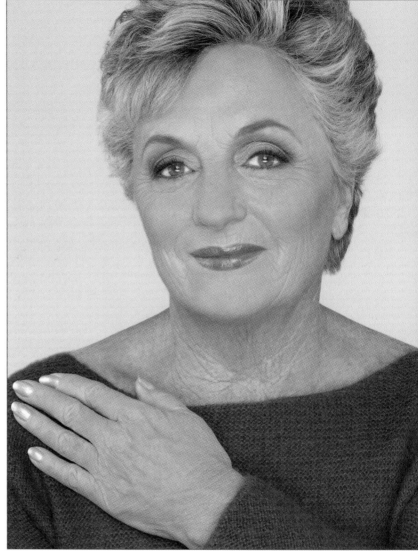

With the makeup on Mary's hands complete, her youthful, energetic look flows from head to toe! Using makeup to cover up age spots—whether they are on your hands, neck, chest, or any other part of your body—works especially well if you're going to a special event or going out for the evening. But it's not for everyday chores such as doing the dishes, changing diapers, or driving the car pool.

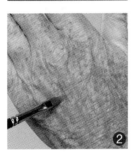

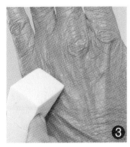

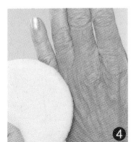

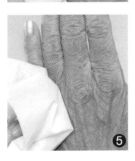

1 While the makeup on Mary's face adequately covers up the age and sun spots there and brings out her youthful beautiful features, the sun spots on her hands are not as smooth and might give away her age. Yet Mary's hands can look as smooth and young as her face, without having to risk laser surgery, dermabrasion, or collagen injections.

2 Using a thin concealer brush, apply a yellow-based concealer over the sun spots. Using the tip of the brush, take a small amount of concealer and apply it on only the larger, most noticeable spots. Blend with the edge of the brush or pat it with your finger. Waterproof concealers and foundations are available in both drugstores and department stores.

3 Using a wedge makeup sponge, apply foundation (there are waterproof ones available) over the top of the hands. Remember the areas between your fingers and around the nails. When applying the foundation, pat it over the concealer instead of rubbing it, so as not to blend anything away. Clean off any excess that might have ended up on your nails or inside the hand.

4 Using a powder puff, dip into loose powder and dab to set the foundation into the hands. When applying the foundation and powder, try blending them into the wrist area, leaving a natural fading of the shades into the arm.

5 With a tissue, blot off any excess powder or oil from the hand until the tissue comes off clean. When you blot, try not to rub off the makeup; simply apply over the area and dab. Again, if any ended up in places you don't need it, just wipe it off with the tissue. It really won't get on your clothes if you properly dab. Clean off your palms and insides of your hands and nails. These steps can be repeated. If you want to really secure it and don't have access to waterproof foundation, just repeat the foundation and dabbing process.

You can use a dual-finish powder with a powder brush instead of foundation and powder. It's a quick fix, and it still needs to be dabbed with a tissue.

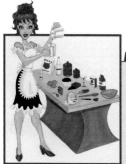

- **Honey and baby oil** combined and rubbed on the body will make it incredibly soft. Be sure to rinse this off before leaving the bath.
- **Milk** will add a smooth texture to the body; try adding some to your next bath.
- **Quick weight-loss tip:** Two garlic tablets and two papaya enzymes before every meal can help you lose up to five pounds in one week.
- **Hair conditioner:** Instead of shaving cream, use hair conditioner to shave your legs. It will leave them silky and smooth as well as saving you a moisturizing step.
- **Sea salt:** Rub over face and body. It will give an invigorating feeling.
- **Baking soda:** For a great, inexpensive exfoliator, mix three-quarters of a cup of baking soda with one-quarter cup of water. Gently rub this on your face for three minutes, then rinse off. Or add about half a box to the bath to soothe itching skin, irritation, or sunburn.
- **Epsom salts** will ease aching muscles and swelling.
- **Lemon juice** will whiten brittle fingernails.
- **Orange slices** added to your bath will provide a natural and easy aromatherapy.
- **Fruit Jell-O** will take away foot odor. Submerge your feet into a cool bucket of prepared Jell-O and enjoy.
- **Lemon, lime, honey, and yogurt** can lighten age and sun spots. Mix the juice from one lemon and one lime with two tablespoons of honey and two ounces of plain yogurt. Massage into spots at least once a week.
- **Lemons and powdered milk** can act as an exfoliator and skin rejuvenator. Mix the juice of two lemons with one cup of powdered milk and enough water to create a thick paste. Let this stand for twenty minutes, and then use the paste to gently massage off dead skin around your knees and elbows. The area will be naturally softened and bleached.
- **Caffeine** is the main ingredient in those expensive cellulite creams. Your regular caffeinated coffee grounds (left over from this morning) can be rubbed into those annoying cellulite areas. Since this can get a bit messy, try doing it in the bathtub or shower.
- **Herbal wraps** are easy to create. For one similar to those offered at expensive spas, mix one cup of corn oil, half a cup of grapefruit juice, and two teaspoons of dried thyme. Work the mixture into the thigh, hip, and butt areas. Cover the areas with plastic wrap, locking in the heat from your body. To accelerate the results, lay a heating pad over the desired areas for several minutes.

Until now, you may have stood helplessly before the mirror wondering how you would ever rid yourself of those blemishes on your skin without resorting to costly and potentially dangerous plastic surgery. Now you know that you really can cover them with makeup! When used wisely, makeup can do the tricks you never thought possible—just look at Mary, Deirdre, and Shirley!

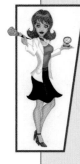

For the Body

- At one time or another, most of us have experienced hickeys, bruises, cuts, or burns. The method for covering the tattoos works the same way to cover any of the above. The shades might change depending on the stage of the bruise or hickey.

- Most of us take care of our face with cleansers and moisturizers yet totally neglect our body—our back and arms, for example. Take the time in the shower to gently exfoliate your body with a loofah or a washcloth. Try some Epsom salts in the bath, which can be used to exfoliate with a washcloth. Apply a body oil or moisturizer to your body before you completely dry off. (This will also help self-tanners go on much smoother.)

- Veins running across the legs or arms can be covered in the same way as the spots and the tattoos. Self-tanners will also help hide bluish veins.

- Use a pumice stone in the bath or shower to keep your feet smooth. They need moisturizing as well.

- Get a pedicure every once in a while. If you can't go to a professional, do it yourself.

- Have a professional massage every now and then. It's great for circulation as well as reducing stress.

- Chubs Baby Wipes are alcohol-free and hypoallergenic. They are great for removing stains from clothes—makeup, deodorant, food, and much more—and dry pretty quickly. This is one of the best things I learned on TV and movie sets.

- If you get a sunburn, take aspirin ASAP to reduce blood flow to the irritated area, and then apply aloe vera gel to soothe the skin.

Tools for Your Body

- Concealer, foundation, loose powder
- Sponge, powder puff
- Brushes: concealer— thin, concealer—thick, powder or blush brush
- Tissue

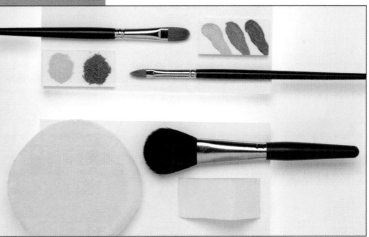

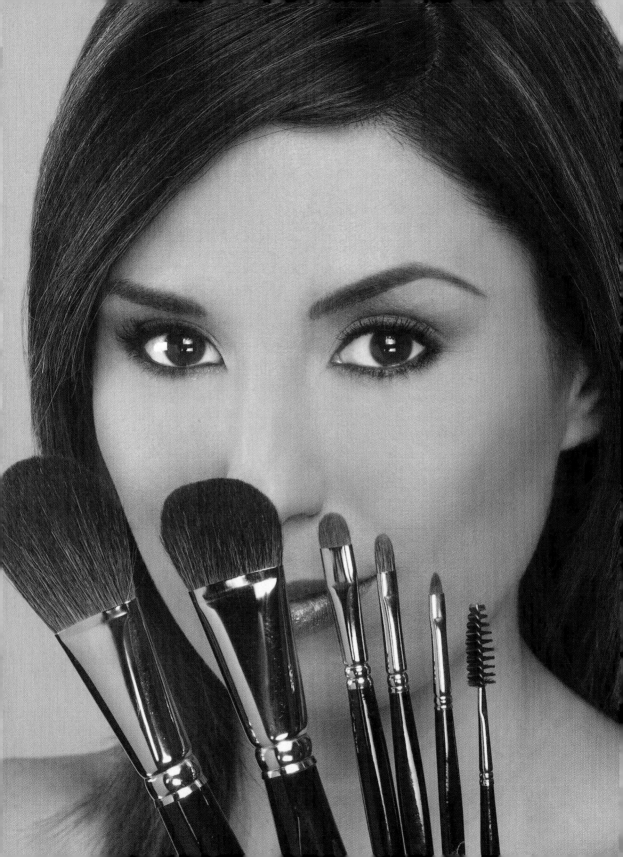

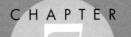
more about the tools of the trade

I t may be hard to believe that you can so totally alter your face, nose, lips, breasts—in short, your whole appearance—simply by using makeup. Next to the invention of tampons, it's perhaps the best secret there is—for women at least (although men sure could take advantage of some of these tricks, too!). The key to transforming yourself into a bodacious Jennifer Lopez one day and a much more understated Annette Bening the next is learning which tools of the trade will really help you transform your face, in whatever way you wish.

Just think of your makeup tools, from the blush brush to the eye curler, as toys for grown-ups—they're fun! In each chapter here, I've provided you with guidelines, but I've also encouraged you to experiment. Play with color; how else will you find out what is right for you? And what suits you one day may not fit your mood the next.

This chapter details all the tools you'll ever need to transform yourself. This is one investment worth making. For example, high-quality brushes might cost a bit more, but with proper care they will last for years and make a big difference in the masterpiece you create on a daily basis. The tools listed here are available at many major drugstores and department stores. Many drugstores now carry high-quality brushes and cosmetics, so make sure you shop around. Most makeup contains basically the same ingredients. When you pay more, you are often paying for the service and packaging—not the product. At times we all like a little more service and an opportunity to try on different shades, textures, and techniques available at the counters. At other times, however, saving money at drugstores is also a good idea for things like mascara, liners, and lip colors. But no matter which brand you buy, you'll still be able to get the job done. Just give it a try!

Your Essential Tools

BRUSHES

There are so many brushes! What are they for and where do you start? Do you buy an entire set or should you buy one at a time? The right brushes will make the difference in getting the effect you want with makeup. You can have the most expensive makeup in the world, but if you don't have the right tools to apply it with, the effect can get lost.

Let me start with this: I do not recommend buying an entire makeup brush set. I will, however, recommend that you select the brushes and tools you need according to the area you want to concentrate on. Remember, many brushes can be used for several different tasks. With proper care, good brushes can last you a very long time. This is an investment worth making. Buy the best you can afford.

Brushes are either natural or synthetic:

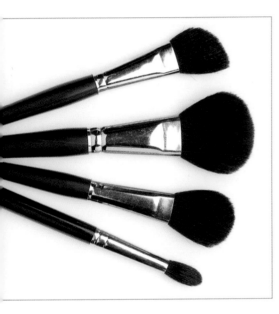

- **Natural bristles**
  Sable and blue squirrel brushes transfer powders from the shadow to the application location best due to their "scaled" hairs, which hold on to powder. These are more costly, but they're also long lasting, soft, and pleasant to the touch and on your skin.

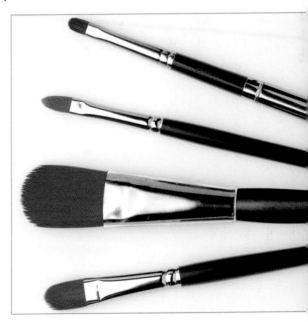

- **Synthetic bristles**
  Work best for applying creams, including concealer, foundation, lipstick, eyeliner, and eyebrow creams. Synthetics are less expensive and can be found in art supply stores as well as drug- and department stores.

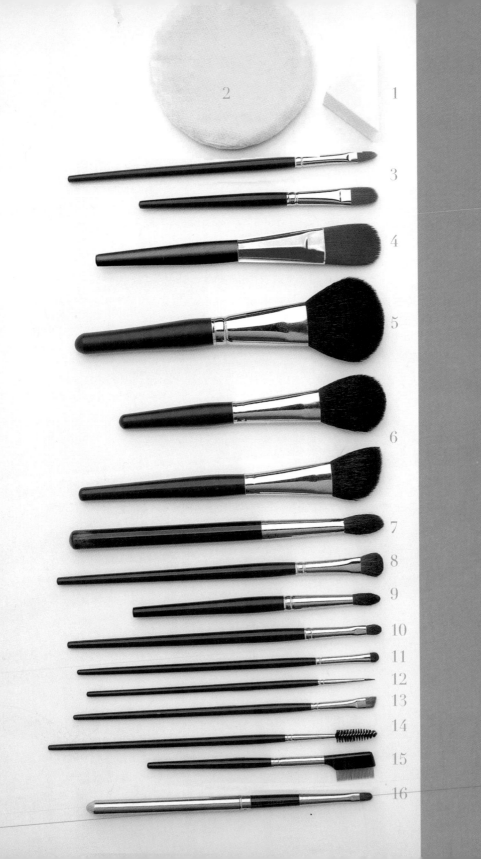

1. Wedge-shaped sponge:

You use the wedge-shaped sponge to apply foundation. Note that it can be used with all foundations—including liquid, cream, stick, and dual finish—and will give you control and help apply the foundation evenly. It can also be used to apply powder to such delicate areas as under the eyes and around the edges of the lips, as well as to apply contouring (shading and highlighting). It is washable and should be one of your makeup bag staples. Sponges should be thrown out after about a week. But don't worry—they're cheap (about $3 a bag of 30) and readily available; both drugstores and department stores sell them.

2. Velour powder puff:

These round puffs should be about the size of your palm and are used with face powder to "seal" the foundation. A puff will give your face a soft sheer appearance and prevent the foundation from moving. It's washable and will last about six months.

3. Concealer brush:

This brush should be made of synthetic material and should be firm and tapered at the end. I suggest you use one thin, narrow brush for spot applications like minor blemishes, as well as one that is slightly thicker for larger areas, such as around the eyes and T-zone.

4. Foundation brush:

This large synthetic brush (a very large version of a concealer brush) is used to apply cream foundation or a cream blush for a smooth, sheer effect.

5. Powder brush:

This is the largest fluffy brush in your kit. It's used to dust face powder lightly over your face to set the foundation. The fuller the brush, the more the powder will be spread out. Try to use this brush only for powder, and avoid using it for blush or bronzing.

6. Blush brush:

You know what this is used for—to accentuate your already gorgeous cheekbones. Try a medium-full round or angled blush brush that is tapered at the sides to allow for controlled application and blending.

7. Long blender blush brush:

This is a thin blush brush used in delicate or hard-to-reach areas, such as under the eyes and between the breasts.

8. Allover eye shadow brush:

When you're shopping for this smaller brush, be sure to look for a full-cut flat brush for applying color *over the entire lid*. It is best used for the light, neutral-toned colors applied all over the lid.

9. Eye blender brush:

A long, fluffy brush tapered at the end. Used in the crease area to blend out the crease and smooth out the contour.

10. Eye definer/contour brush:

A medium-narrow brush that's tapered at the end and slightly firm for good control. This brush will give precise control to create the contours to define the crease of the eye.

11. Eye smudger brush:

A short, firm brush tapered at the edges will give you control of applying color at precise areas. This will be your smoke-out brush.

12. Eyeliner brush:

A small, very thin, firm, narrow brush used to line the eyes with a liquid or cream liner. This brush is also available in art supply stores (and much cheaper there).

13. Eyebrow brush:

A brush with firm bristles clipped at an angle to apply shadow to your brows. It will add the finishing touch to the eye.

14. Spooly:

This small brush looks like a mascara brush and can be used either to brush up brow hair or to remove excess mascara.

15. Eyelash separator comb:

If your lashes get stuck together or clumpy after you apply mascara, use a fine-toothed comb to carefully brush through them before the mascara dries.

16. Lip brush:

A small, firm, narrow brush tapered for better control and to keep lipstick on longer, as well as prevent it from smudging onto your face.

17. False lashes:

For special occasions, full or individual lashes can make that subtle difference. Totally worth the effort.

18. Eyelash glue:

Is available in clear and in black. I prefer the waterproof type. First, apply the glue, then let it stand for fifteen to thirty seconds before applying the lashes. Eyelash glue can also be used to apply accessories such as rhinestones to the eyes or face.

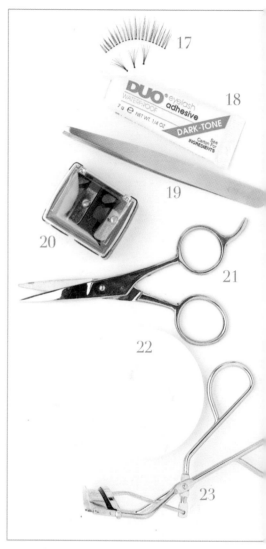

19. **Tweezers:**

The good-quality angled metal ones are best for precision and durability. They're good not only for plucking unwanted hairs but also for placing and applying false lashes. (I recommend using an old pair for the lashes.)

20. **Pencil sharpener:**

To keep all pencils sharp for best application.

21. **Scissors:**

Just in case—to trim eyebrow hairs, false lashes, unwanted facial hair, and so on.

22. **Cream bleach:**

Use to bleach and lighten the eyebrows or any other facial hair. Leave on for five to fifteen minutes, depending on the original shade of your hair and your skin sensitivity.

23. **Eyelash curler:**

I highly recommend curling your lashes *before* applying mascara. Take the curler and place it almost at the base of the lashes. Squeeze a few times while moving it outward to the end of the lashes, squeezing as you go. This will look like a natural curl. (*Tip:* You can heat a metal curler with a hair dryer or simply by placing the tip on a lightbulb. Make sure it does not get too hot. The effect will be much like that of a curling iron on your hair.)

More Tools

- **Eyebrow stencils:**
Stencils come in many shapes. They make shaping the brows easier. They are reversible: Simply wipe off one side before flipping over to the other. Just place and fill in with powder, using an eyebrow brush and a powdered shadow.

- **Brush cleaner:**
Although expensive cleaners are available on the market, I recommend simply using your shampoo. Wash your brushes once a week with shampoo or even a mild soap. Get a good lather going and rotate around your palm. Rinse thoroughly, squeeze out any excess water with your hand, and lay flat to dry. Once a month, you can even use conditioner. In this case, either let the hairs dry on the edge of a table or place them somewhere that air can circulate through. Avoid drying the brushes flat on a towel, for this can leave behind an odor, and the brush might dry in an awkward shape.

- **Q-tips:**
Great for fast and easy cleanups, blending, and even applying color in a pinch.

- **Cotton balls or puffs:**
Use to remove makeup and apply toner or astringent.

- **Fingers:**
Your most trusted tool. You can apply everything with them (so you don't have an excuse when you forget your kit!). The heat in your fingers will help melt a thick concealer into place (especially under the eyes). You can also use them to blend cream blushes, or to apply lip balm or gloss. Don't forget to clean your hands when going from one application or color to another.

The Makeup

The weather changes every day, and so do our moods. How can we expect our skin and makeup needs to be the same? Some days we might need a light extra moisturizer when our skin seems especially dry. On other days, we may need a touch of deeper concealer when an uninvited blemish shows up. Maybe that last cocktail didn't help your puffiness, or getting in at 3 A.M. added to the intensity of those undereye circles.

My goal in this book is to give you choices and show you my techniques for combating the unsightly effects of lack of sleep, too much sugar, or too much fun! Instead of rules, in other words, I give you options. Then you can become the makeup artist. I hope you will learn how to appreciate and admire your face—after all, it is your greatest canvas. The palette of colors is not as vital as the techniques and placement.

You would think that all the choices women now have for makeup would make life easier. I'm not sure about that. It seems to me that at times it can be even more confusing. Too many choices seem to feel a bit intimidating and confusing. A question I hear often is, "Should I buy my makeup in a department store or a drugstore?" Before I answer that question, let me ask you, "Do you buy all your clothes at a department store?" Some of the wealthiest women I know buy some things at the most expensive department stores and others at the dollar store. The key is knowing what to pay extra for, what to save money on, and how to put it together while making it all look like it's the best. The same companies own many of the most familiar department-store and drugstore cosmetics. They even manufacture them in the same plants. Some are just packaged beautifully for department stores (sometimes with added perfumes), others more simply for drugstores. The basic ingredients are almost identical.

In my opinion, the best thing about shopping in a department store is the fact that you get waited on and can try out all the different fun makeup shades, textures, techniques, and trends. While you're there, you might even want to get a makeover and possibly learn a few new styles for your makeup application. Just be aware that the salesperson is giving you her time for a reason: to make a sale. So, although most salespeople do not work on commission, they still want to sell you as much product as they can. In the end, that free makeover might end up costing you several hundred dollars in products you might not really need or want.

Take your time, and do not make impulse purchases. A very wise and wealthy woman once told me to always wait three days before purchasing anything. If you still want it, then go ahead and get it. If you've moved on to other things, you really didn't need it. Three days may be a bit excessive, but try stepping away from the makeup counter for at least half an hour to think about your potential purchase. If you still need to have that product, then go back and get it.

Products to Look for in a Department Store

- **Foundation:**
  This is a good place to test different shades and textures to see what best suits your skin. Also, it is easy to return or exchange foundation if you find after using it that it doesn't agree with you.
- **Brushes:**
  This is the one item I would recommend researching and spending money on. When shopping for brushes, check their texture, quality, and feel. If your brushes are not good, even the most expensive makeup will not be applied well. I did a spot on TV once in which makeup products from drugstores and department stores were compared. We used two sets of twins (a young set in their early twenties and an older set in their late forties). I used all drugstore makeup, while a different makeup artist used all department-store makeup. When asked to pick out the twins wearing the drugstore makeup, both times the hosts got it wrong. They all picked the twins with the drugstore makeup as wearing the expensive makeup. I made sure to point out that the difference in the way the women looked was all in the application. You can't apply well if your brushes don't work properly. Try them out; test them on the area you're going to use them. Don't impulse-buy brushes you don't need or won't use.

Products to Look for in a Drugstore

Remember, you don't always have to spend a lot of money to get good quality. Also, many drugstores will let you return or exchange makeup you are unhappy with.

- **Mascara:** Try L'Oréal's Architect or Maybelline's Great Lash.
- **Lip liners:** Try Wet & Wild's #666. I still use it today. It's a staple in many makeup artists' kits.
- **Eyeliners:** Any drugstore version will do. These are available in a creamy stick and a pencil. The textures may vary a bit, so find those that suit you best.
- **Lipstick:** They are available in an assortment of colors, textures, and durability. A great way to experiment with new colors without spending a fortune.
- **Lip gloss:** You can find anything from a simple clear gloss to ones filled with shimmers in an assortment of colors.
- **Blush:** Many drugstore brands have a good variety of colors and textures (powder, cream, stick). You might, however, need to try out several until you find the right shade for you.
- **Eye shadow:** You will find a variety of shades and textures (powder, cream, tube, cream pencil). You might need to test out several different brands until you find the colors and textures that best suit you.
- **Face powder:** This comes both pressed and loose. You should try to feel the texture of powders. It might take several tries until you find one that will blend well with your skin.
- **Face moisturizers:** Roc is comparable to expensive doctors' moisturizers that contain fish oils and are quite expensive. Lubriderm lotion works on both face and body. It is also available in SPF (sun protection factor) 15.
- **Body moisturizers:** Nivea or Vaseline body lotions always do the trick.
- **Aquaphor** is the best thing since Vaseline. I use this healing ointment on everything from lips to cuticles, burns, and chapped hands. It's like Vaseline, with an added healing ingredient.
- **Cetaphil Facial Cleanser** is very gentle and removes makeup without causing irritation to the skin.

What follow are lists of the many makeup products available to you—from foundation textures to mascara—and the varieties they come in. Once again, I encourage you to experiment and find out what best suits you on any given day. Have fun with this!

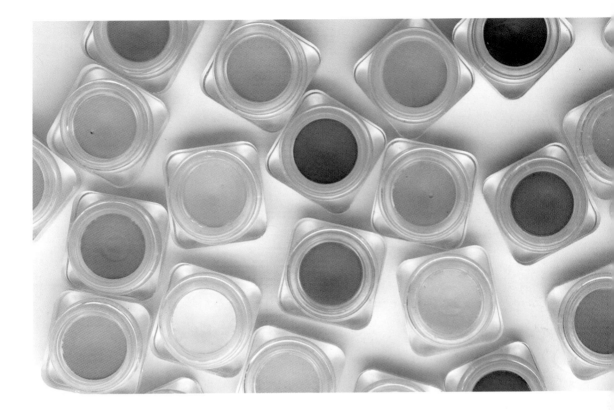

FOUNDATION

In chapter 1, you learned about your specific skin tone and how to choose the right color foundation for you. Many different foundation textures are also available, however. Here's some information that will help you determine which product is most suitable to your needs. Again, your needs will vary according to the season, your mood, and your lifestyle. Remember, the important thing in makeup is finding the shade, intensity, and texture that best suit you.

- **Liquid (sheer):**
This type of foundation is the most commonly used for basic sheer, natural coverage and a simple way to even out skin tone.
- **Cream:**
You can achieve very good coverage with a cream foundation and, depending on your needs, can apply it as sheer or as thick as you desire.
- **Oil-based:**
Use an oil-based foundation if you have very dry skin.
- **Oil-free:**
Since oil-free foundation dries quickly, apply it sparingly and with a sponge.
- **Light reflecting:**
This type of foundation creates a dewy, slightly shimmery effect, and is very good for dry skin.
- **Dual finish:**
This type of foundation is a dry powder or has a wet-to-dry finish. It can be applied with a brush for light coverage or a sponge for thicker coverage.
- **Corrective or highlighter stick:**
It's part foundation, part concealer and works great for quick touch-ups. But, since it catches the light, it can make a feature appear more prominent.
- **Tinted moisturizer:**
This product is good if you have a suntan, or if you are a minimalist and prefer not to use foundation.
- **Anti-shine:**
It's not a foundation, but a gel that will dry up areas prone to being oily or shiny. Be careful when applying it; since it goes on clear, you might apply too much, and then your foundation will get blotchy. You can also use this product on the scalp to eliminate shine.
- **Primer:**
This one extra step will help your foundation and makeup stay on your face. Primer is particularly good for oily skin. If you apply it to your eyelids, it will help prevent creasing.
- **Wrinkle tightener:**
This product comes in a cream or a gel and will help tighten the skin prior to applying foundation. After applying, let it sit for a couple of minutes to become fully absorbed and dry before applying makeup.
- **Cream sticks:**
These foundation products are quite versatile and easy to apply, and they provide good coverage.

CONCEALERS AND HIGHLIGHTERS

Concealer is the key to good coverage. It's available in many variations, including waterproof, and is more opaque and longer lasting than foundation. At times, a concealer might feel a bit thick or dry. You can thin it out by mixing it with either water, a moisturizer, or a foundation. Some women can simply use a concealer as foundation, applying it with a thin brush for spot applications. Because of its opaqueness and thick quality, women who have raised freckles or scars may want to use concealer as an allover foundation. Learning to use concealer properly will make your makeup application a breeze. It can also be used as a primer on lids to help the eye makeup stay on longer.

- **Cream:**
  This is the most versatile and durable, though it can get a bit thick or dry. Also available in waterproof.
- **Pen or twist-up:**
  Use the pen or twist-up concealer for easy application and for quick touch-ups.
- **Tube:**
  This type is more sheer than the rest, and best for using as foundation.
- **Stick:**
  In stick form, concealer is quite versatile and available in both drugstores and department stores.

Remember, all products can be thinned out with moisturizer, foundation, water, or by using your finger to gently pat or rub them.

Shelf Life for Makeup

- Liquid and cream products, including cream foundation, rouge, bronzer, eye shadow, contour, and highlighter: one year.
- All powder products, including loose powder, pressed powder, blush, contour, and eye shadow: two years.
- Mascara and liquid eyeliner: six months.
- Eye pencils, brow pencils, and lip pencils: three years.
- Lipstick, lip color in pots, lip gloss: two years.

To prolong makeup's life, keep items stored in a cool, dry place away from direct sunlight. Capping products tightly after use helps further extend the life of your makeup. Some products benefit from being manufactured with fresh plant extracts, making them more perishable than other brands. These products often have a "use by" date printed on the label.

POWDER

Powder is terrific for setting foundations, absorbing oil, and creating a flawless finish. The following list details the various forms of powder and their uses:

- **Loose/translucent:** Loose powder should feel like silk to the touch. Stay with shades lighter than your own skin tone.
- **Pressed:** Pressed powder or a compact makes a good travel companion for quick touch-ups and when you need to use a mirror.
- **Shimmery:** To achieve a dewy look, shimmery powder can be applied on the face as well as the chest, arms, or anywhere else you might want a little extra shine. It can also be mixed with eye shadows and blushes for some extra glow.
- **Bronzing:** For a healthy look, avoid brushing this all over your face. It may look ruddy. Apply to cheeks, forehead, chin, and eyelids in a quick dusting. Don't forget your chest.

EVE'S TIPS

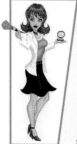

For Powders

- Pump brushes both empty and filled are now readily available. They are great for travel. Just pump and brush it on.
- Once thought of as cakey and heavy, powder is now used to set and maintain a foundation. It can be applied lightly and look translucent. Applied with a powder puff, powder secures the foundation; applied with a brush, it gives a slightly sheer finish. It will keep your foundation in place, help it last longer, and and prevent it from getting on your clothes—or his.
- It's a myth that powder will accentuate the lines around the eyes. Actually, when applied with a puff or lightly dusted with a brush, powder creates a softer look, eliminates shine, and keeps any concealer or foundation from creasing and accentuating lines around the eyes.

The Purpose of Powder

- Applied lightly under the eyes, it can catch any loose eye makeup that might scatter during application. Once you're finished, don't forget to dust off any remains.
- Powder can set lipstick in place and prevent feathering and lipstick bleeding.
- Use it on your scalp to help dry up excess oils.
- On your scalp, it can also fill in areas where the hair is thinning and even cover up any premature roots.
- Powder applied over your foundation will keep the makeup in place much longer.

SHADOWS FOR THE EYES AND CHEEKS

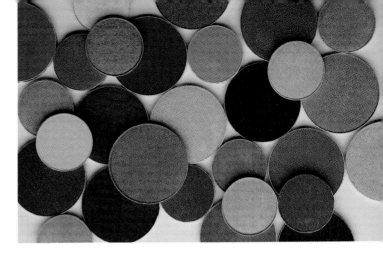

Shadows are simply shades of colors. Much more versatile than you may realize, shadows can be used on any area of the face you choose. You can use cheek colors on your eyes, and vice versa. You might, however, want to avoid using that blue shadow on your cheeks! Usually blush shades are great for the eyes as well. The key is to find good-quality shadows. Look for the intensity of the pigment; you want the color you see to be the color you get when applied. Check that the texture is smooth and able to be blended. The drier your skin, the creamier your makeup should be. Here is a simple guide to the various forms of shadows for your cheeks and eyes.

- Rouge and swivel-up cheek color sticks are great for dry complexions.
- Gel and liquid cheek colors work well for normal skin. Apply with your fingers, a foundation brush, or a sponge to give a subtle natural look. These can be more difficult to control, however, and can appear a bit blotchy if not blended quickly. Effective application requires practice.
- Brush-on blush, which can be used successfully on all skin types, is a must for oily skin, and will help reduce shine on the complexion.
- Shadows come in matte or shimmer finish. The matte shadows last longer and are more natural looking. When using shimmers, I prefer to apply them over a matte shadow; it helps the shimmers last longer.
- On eyelids, shadow can be applied wet or dry.
- A taupe eye shadow will work great as a contour around the cheeks and to fill in the eyebrows as well as fill in any hair that might be thinning or need a touch-up.
- An allover light shadow can be used as a highlighter on your upper cheekbone as well as your forehead.

Again, it's your palette; be versatile and creative!

Natural Blush

Blood vessels lie directly under the skin. When we're aroused, embarrassed, excited, or active, these blood vessels enlarge, allowing a greater amount of blood to flow to the skin. The result of this is visible as flushed cheeks.

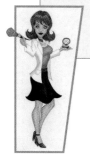

You can use your favorite lipstick color as a cream blush.

MASCARA

Mascara is one of those products that don't vary much in quality—regardless of whether you pay $22 or $3.99. Here is what you need to know:

- Mascara comes in two varieties: regular and waterproof.
- It also addresses several needs, particularly lengthening, thickening, and conditioning the eyelashes.
- The waterproof type has long-lasting power through water and tears, but it may be a bit drying.
- Clear mascara is used to moisturize and add shine to lashes. It's for the natural look and the minimalist.
- Mascara now is available in many shades, including clear.
- For the most dramatic effect, I prefer using black mascara. I use brown for young people or for that very natural look.

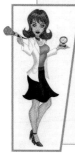

For Mascara

- To prevent mascara from clumping, dab a tissue around the wand and remove excess color prior to applying.
- Avoid pumping the mascara brush in and out of the tube. This will only let air into the tube and dry out the mascara. Try rotating the wand in a circular motion and pulling it out.

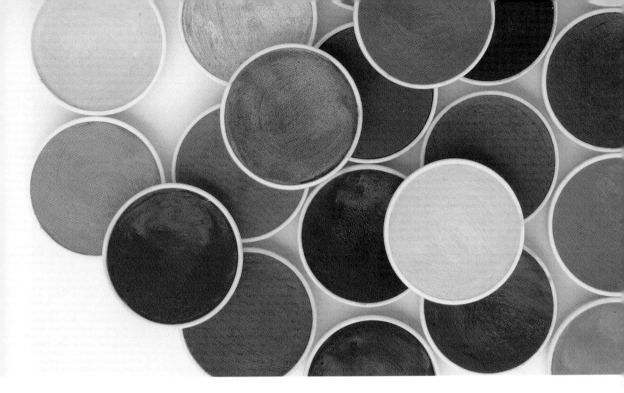

LIPSTICK AND GLOSS

Lips become flushed and rosy when we're sexually aroused. We wear lip color to mimic this effect.

- **Cream:**

  This is the most common type of lip color. It provides good creamy coverage while going on smooth and moisturizing lips.
- **Matte:**

  For the most coverage. It provides a flat matte finish that stays on, but can be a bit drying.
- **Sheer:**

  Light, subtle coverage that's good for a natural look.
- **All day/long wearing:**

  Long-lasting lip colors provide good coverage. Most are drying but come with a protective moisturizing top coat. They are not very blendable and can cake up when reapplied. With practice, however, they can keep your daily lipstick application to a minimum.
- **Gloss:**

  Good for applying alone for a quick, natural shine or to top off a lipstick to give dimension and make your lips "pop."

PENCILS FOR THE LIPS AND EYES

Pencils provide you with an indispensable way to accentuate and add contour and dimension to your lips. Around the eyes, they help bring dramatic attention to one of your most powerful features.

- Pencil liner comes in four types: creamy, twist-up, waterproof, and smokers.
- Liquid or pen liner is applied with the tip of the product and produces the most intense line. Try out the product on the back of your hand to check the amount of liquid. This will take a bit of practice. Try to apply powder over a liquid to set it.
- Eyeliner comes in pencil or liquid forms, or as a powder that you can apply with an eyeliner brush. You can also choose among products that are creamy, smooth, waterproof, and retractable.
- Eyeliner should be soft to glide on smoothly yet firm for good control.

Regardless of which type you use, apply the product as close to the lash line as possible.

Now you have all the tools and tips you need to know how to make your beautiful self the most knockout gorgeous you can be. As you can see, taking just a little bit of time to apply makeup correctly, with the aid of a few handy-dandy tools, can allow you to do your own makeover at home without paying a professional. And the best part is, you're going to enjoy yourself. It will feel liberating to see those undereye circles magically disappear. Or those eyebrows shaped, or lips plumped! By using makeup, you have the ability to transform your features and accentuate the beautiful face you already have. Have fun, and enjoy the new you!

EVE PEARL is a three-time Emmy Award–winning celebrity makeup artist who has more than fifteen years' experience in TV, theater, print, and film. She is currently the key makeup artist on ABC's *The View*, where she also does on-air segments performing makeovers and giving makeup tips. Her credits include "The Academy Awards," *The Today Show, Live with Regis & Kelly,* American Ballet Theatre, Metropolitan Opera, *Who Wants to Be a Millionaire?, The Tonight Show with Jay Leno, All My Children,* and *Saturday Night Live.* Her work has appeared in magazines such as *InStyle, Vanity Fair, Good Housekeeping, More People, Ladies' Home Journal, Prevention,* and *TV Guide.* She's also worked on numerous celebrities, including Brooke Shields, Kelly Ripa, Al Pacino, Mira Sorvino, Barbara Walters, and Liza Minnelli. Eve currently resides in New York City with her family.

Visit Eve Pearl at www.evepearl.com or www.greatfaces.com.